Making the Most of Your Medical Career

MAXIMISING YOUR CHANCES OF SUCCESS

DR DAVID McGOWAN

Core Surgical Trainee
Northern General Hospital
Sheffield

and

DR HELEN SIMS

Specialty Medical Trainee and Teaching Fellow
Royal United Hospital
Bath

Foreword by
DR INAM HAQ
Director of Undergraduate Studies
Reader in Medical Education and Rheumatology
Brighton and Sussex Medical School
University of Brighton

Radcliffe Publishing
London • New York

Radcliffe Publishing Ltd
St Mark's House
Shepherdess Walk
London N1 7BQ
United Kingdom

www.radcliffehealth.com

British Library Cataloguing in Publication Data

A catalogue record for this book is available from the British Library.

ISBN-13: 978 184619 975 2

The paper used for the text pages of this book is FSC® certified. FSC (The Forest Stewardship Council®) is an international network to promote responsible management of the world's forests.

Typeset by Darkriver Design, Auckland, New Zealand
Manufacturing managed by 21six

Contents

Preface

The majority of medical careers are becoming increasingly competitive, with many specialties subject to competition ratios of over 10 applicants for each place. The need for medical students, Foundation trainees and those in core training to be aware of the many challenges that lie ahead is obvious, as these are the people who are still to undertake an application that is subject to this increasingly competitive world. The importance of understanding what lies ahead and how to best prepare for this is something that cannot be understated. Preparation for your higher specialty training applications can begin as soon as you start medical school or can start as late as your second core training year. The differences in what can be achieved between these two approaches should be obvious to anyone. We hope that by reading this book not only will people be motivated to start developing their personal portfolio sooner, but also that they are able to address the whole spectrum of what it is that they will be assessed on when applying for jobs.

This book is by no means a step-by-step guide of how to get the perfect curriculum vitae (CV), for there are many books much longer than this that look at each individual aspect of a medical CV. Nor does this book promise to offer secrets that are not already known by many people.

This book aims to educate the reader in two very important areas: first, this book will act as a source of information on all aspects of medical careers and job applications, acting as a reference point for those wanting to optimise their chances of success, utilising the knowledge garnered from myriad written sources and experts to ensure complete appreciation of the topic; second, it will act to retrain the way you look at your working life, introducing you to ideas of how to identify opportunities to improve your CV in situations that are normally not seen as an opportunity or which are even seen as a burden. As an example, all Foundation year trainees undertake audits, yet the majority do not attempt to complete the audit cycle – that is, re-audit after their recommendations have been implemented. Furthermore, even fewer audits are written up and submitted to peer-reviewed journals for publication. This is not to say that *every* audit is suitable for publication, but if you don't try you will never know.

Herein lies the main overriding aim of this book: to change how you see the clinical world. If you see it as a means to work and get paid and do not undertake any 'extracurricular activities', then you should be prepared for an uphill struggle when applying for future career posts. If you embrace this aspect of the medical career ladder, then you will almost certainly improve your chances in landing your future job and you may also find that you enjoy the challenges and rewards of undertaking these endeavours.

Medical careers have changed and getting through applications to jobs is as much about learning how to play the game as it is about being the best in your field. This may be seen as a sad fact, but it is the case as things stand, so think of the old adage *'if you fail to prepare, prepare to fail'*. When reading this book, appreciate the general lessons on how to approach each section of your career – medical school, Foundation training and core training – from the early chapters; use the MARKET approach towards developing your portfolio; and use the latter stages to help with the intricacies of the individual challenges that you will face. By doing this you will soon observe that you are developing a well-rounded CV as well as discovering many new and exciting opportunities along the way.

David McGowan
Helen Sims
June 2014

Foreword

I am delighted to write the foreword for this book. It is certainly something I wish I had had during my training!

It provides an excellent and easy-to-read path to making the most of your medical career starting as a student. I think it is realistic in that it advocates a good mix between work, rest and play.

I was particularly pleased to see that education and teaching is mentioned as a domain in which students should get further experience as I think this will be increasingly required as part of undergraduate and postgraduate training.

Research is an area that as a student often seems quite difficult to navigate, and the authors have provided a really sensible way of getting into research, whatever your field of interest.

This book provides a ready source of really useful hints and tips that will help anyone reading this book maximise their personal and professional development. I am also very proud to see so many of our ex-Brighton and Sussex Medical School students as authors in this book.

Dr Inam Haq
Director of Undergraduate Studies
Reader in Medical Education and Rheumatology
Brighton and Sussex Medical School
University of Brighton
June 2014

About the authors

David McGowan
David attended the University of Southampton from 2003 to 2007, reading audiology, and then attended Brighton and Sussex Medical School between 2007 and 2012, graduating with honours in obstetrics and gynaecology, paediatrics and surgery. David is continuing his training in surgery in the Northern Deanery while pursuing his ambition of training in cardiothoracic surgery. David is the author of two research papers, four case reports, and 12 communication and discussion articles. These have been published in multiple journals including the *Lancet* and the *BMJ*.

Helen Sims
Helen graduated from the International School Basel in 2006 and attended Brighton and Sussex Medical School, graduating with a distinction and honours in obstetrics and gynaecology, paediatrics and surgery. Helen has since worked as a Foundation Year 1 doctor at the Gloucestershire Royal Hospital and as a Foundation Year 2 doctor at the Royal United Hospital Bath. Helen is pursuing her ambition of working in medicine and is undertaking a teaching fellowship year prior to undertaking her core medical training. Helen has authored one research paper and three communication and discussion articles.

List of contributors

Dr Nerys Conway
Specialty Trainee Year 5, Acute Internal
Medicine
Severn Deanery
National Trainee Representative for
Society of Acute Medicine

Mr Mark Cookson
Specialty Trainee Year 7 Trauma &
Orthopaedics
London Deanery, SE Thames Rotation

Dr Samantha Fossey
Core Surgical Trainee Year 2, General
Surgery
Kent, Surrey and Sussex Deanery

Mr Michael Ghosh-Dastidar
Specialty Trainee Year 5 Cardiothoracic
Surgery
London Deanery

Dr Liam Gillespie
Core Surgical Trainee Year 2
North Western Deanery
Academic Leadership Trainee

Dr Lyudmila Kishikova
Foundation Year 2 Doctor
Peninsula Deanery

Dr Meher Lad
Specialty Trainee Year 1 Academic
Clinical Fellow, Neurology
Northern Deanery

Dr Nigel Mabvuure
Foundation Year 2 Doctor
Academic Foundation Trainee in Plastic
Surgery
Scotland Deanery

Dr Guy Mole
Core Surgical Trainee Year 2
London Deanery
Academic Management and Leadership
Foundation Trainee

Dr Joseph M Norris
Foundation Year 2 Doctor
Academic Foundation Trainee in
Surgery
Cambridge Deanery

Dr Matthew Smith
Foundation Year 2 Doctor
Peninsula Deanery

Dr Natalie Smith
Core Trainee Year 2, Anaesthetics and
Intensive Care Medicine
Wessex Deanery

Mr Charles Zammit
*Consultant Breast and Endocrine
Surgeon
Brighton and Sussex University
Hospitals NHS Trust*

Section 1

Medical careers and the training pathway

The scope of medical careers is vast, and limited almost only by your imagination. Most people tend to think of a few of the main specialties – anaesthetics, general practice, medicine, paediatrics or surgery. However, within these, and also outside of them, there are myriad careers available to you – from audiological medicine to orthopaedic surgery, histopathology to public health. The nuances of the individual careers are beyond the scope of this book, but this section will help summarise the main differences among the career pathways.

The first chapter of this book will cover the structure of the main career pathways, while the second will cover the points at which there is competition within the career pathways of the main specialties.

These chapters aim to provide you with the knowledge necessary to ensure you are aware and prepared for any application and to make sure you understand the basic career structure. This knowledge is subject to change almost perpetually, but the main aspects of this will remain the same – once you are in medical school you will need to apply for Foundation training; once in Foundation training you will need to apply for core or specialty training; if you go through core training, you will need to apply for specialty training; and once in specialty training, you will need to apply for consultancy posts. Knowing about this allows you to prepare for the next application, and enables you to show yourself in the best light in the application process.

CHAPTER 1

Your medical career

Medical careers are almost as diverse as your imagination. Everyone knows that doctors work in hospitals, general practice and laboratories, but not everyone knows that there are many, sometimes (if you are lucky) exotic, careers to be had in medicine, ranging from a cruise ship doctor to a prison physician, from the doctor to the England football team to working on mercy ships providing healthcare relief in deprived countries. What you want to do with your career depends on one person: *you*. This is something of utmost importance to appreciate – you are only required to do what you want to do.

A medical career does not start as you begin your Foundation Year 1 post in your first role as a doctor, nor does it begin once you move into specialist training. It has a more humble origin: your first day of medical school. It is here that you are classed as a 'medical professional', your behaviour can result in you not passing to become a doctor and your actions can have a huge bearing on your future career.

Starting your first day of medical school, the last thing you envisage is this being the first day of your long career as a doctor, as you may see yourself as a student. However, as of day one you are a medical professional, with all of the associated expectations in terms of behaviour and professionalism. It is here that your experiences can truly change who and what you want to become. This is also the only time in your career that you will have as much free time to dedicate to improving your future chances in your career.

It is pertinent here to state it is vital that you are aware of the great adage *'all work and no play makes Jack a dull boy!'* Nowhere is this truer than when undertaking what is possibly the toughest and most demanding degree of them all, followed by one of the toughest and most demanding (and also greatly rewarding) careers.

So, what do you have to do? Well, first of all, remain yourself. You are your greatest asset and who you are is something that should be embraced, not resisted. It should be the foundation upon which you build your (professional) castle. Remaining 'you' not only allows you to make the most of your natural talents and avoid your shortcomings but also enables you to lead as rich, fulfilling and diverse a life as you possibly can.

Then you need to understand where you are going. The specific career pathway of the profession you ultimately end up pursuing is always going to vary slightly from all others, but there is a rough generic training pathway outline. You start as a medical student, you graduate and become a Foundation doctor, then you move on to become a 'core trainee', followed by specialist training. Then you obtain your Certificate of Completion of Training and can become a general practice partner, consultant or another of the myriad positions available to those with a medical background.

Knowing this general structure of what is ahead, and appreciating where you are going to be 'in competition' with others – that is, there are more people applying for jobs than there are posts available – will hold you in good stead for the future.

The basic structure of each stage of the medical career is briefly described as follows.

Medical school: 4–6 years where you are a student and learn all of the skills necessary to become a safe and competent doctor. This is a place where you will have great opportunities to explore the direction in which you want your future career to go. It is also the one place where failing examinations can mean you are no longer a doctor, so take care and make sure medical school examinations come before extracurricular activities.

Foundation training: 2 years straight after medical school. Here you take your medical school teaching and sculpt it into something that takes you from simply being safe and competent to becoming an effective, knowledgeable and productive member of the team. *See* Chapter 4 if you wish to read more about Foundation training.

Core training (or Specialty Training Years 1 and 2 (ST1 and ST2) of run-through training): 2 further years of learning how to be even more knowledgeable and productive in a specific area of medicine. Here you will have 'nailed your colours to the mast' in terms of what it is you want to do with your career, be it general practice, acute medicine or general surgery. Here you will be able to begin your learning of the finer and more difficult aspects of your chosen career path and learn to become a team leader capable of making complex medical decisions regarding patients. For some specialties it is necessary to have completed your membership examinations prior to graduating from this stage of training. Further information regarding this stage of your career can be found in Chapter 5.

Specialty training: 4–7 years of training, from Specialty Training Years 3 or 4 (ST3 or ST4) onwards, where you learn the specific skills and knowledge so that you are able to become a consultant in your chosen career area. You also need to learn much alongside your clinical knowledge – how to be a leader of the team, how to make sometimes difficult decisions, how to organise your time among many different schedules (outpatient clinics, administrative tasks, ward work, and so forth). For more information on specialty training, *see* Chapter 6.

Academic training: this can involve all or part of the academic training pathway. This is the route by which you should travel if you are more interested in academic work and becoming involved with university teaching. Further details can be found in Chapter 7.

Most differences in training pathways are among the main branches of medical careers – medicine, surgery, general practice, anaesthetics, paediatrics, pathology, and so forth. With these different training pathways come different examinations (*see* Chapter 14, 'K: knowledge') and different requirements of the trainees.

COMPETITION

Competition is a semi-dirty word in medicine. We are all colleagues, we are not 'against' one another, and we are all working together for the benefit of our patients. However, at certain times in your career, there are points when your attainment of your ambition of becoming a trainee in a certain career pathway is going to depend on your application and interview being better than the other applicants.

Where does this competition arise? Well, this is difficult to say for each career pathway but, basically, when you change job titles, you can safely bet you will have had some form of application, and thus competition, to get there. Medical student to Foundation doctor, Foundation doctor to core trainee, core trainee to specialist trainee, these all require applications and competition (*see* Figure 1.1).

SUMMARY

It is easy to see that with such diverse career pathways and different methods of reaching what you want to do, it is not possible for any book smaller than a small house to have a step-by-step guide on how to achieve your career ambitions! Saying, 'do X, Y and Z and you will become a consultant in your chosen career' is impossible, as there are no such rules. It is more important to be aware of what awaits you – where is the competition, when do I need to be preparing for an application, what are the general areas that I need to be working on to address my limitations and improve my application? While it is not possible to say that doing specific things will get you a job, doing the basics and covering all of your bases will usually be enough to get you into the interview room and, with a little preparation, you will succeed in that and then you will be onto the next step of this fabulous journey.

There are simple messages that are found throughout this book: be aware of what is in front of you – forewarned is forearmed; do not become amazing in one area of your development to the detriment of all others – there is no point having 10 peer-reviewed research papers if you have no audits or teaching experience, or you have not sat postgraduate examinations or been on any extracurricular courses. Being average in all subject areas will score you more highly in applications and it will also lead to you being a well-rounded doctor with a greater skill set to utilise in your daily life. However, and this is the most important message of the entire book: do not work too hard, and make sure you enjoy yourself – there is no point in becoming professor of medicine if you do not gain pleasure on a day-to-day basis. The most successful person in the world is the one who smiles the most!

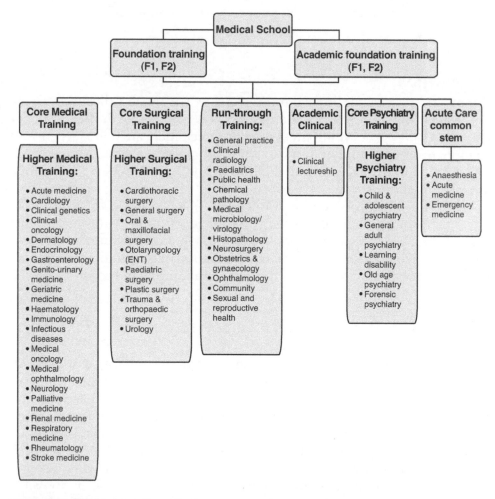

FIGURE 1.1 Different training pathways

CHAPTER 2

The training pathways: what you need to be doing and by when

Dr Lyudmila Kishikova

Understanding how postgraduate training pathways are organised is very important, and possessing such knowledge is vital in improving your chances of a successful career. This acts as a motivating factor for many an individual when beginning to strategically plan what is needed for the competitive stages of his or her career pathway. A considerable number of people lack this knowledge and so blindly send off applications for very competitive training posts. Knowing *what* you need to do is the first step in reaching your career goals, which this book will attempt to convey. However, equally important is knowing *when* you need to have achieved certain things; having a concrete deadline allows you to organise yourself most effectively.

This chapter is intended to familiarise you with the UK postgraduate training pathways, the prerequisites required for each and what you need to achieve and when.

START TO DEVELOP YOUR CURRICULUM VITAE WHILE AT MEDICAL SCHOOL

Entrance to all training pathways requires an appropriate medical degree and the completion of the 2 Foundation years. Regardless of this, it is preferable to have a rough idea as to which training pathway you are hoping to take *before* completing medical school. Unless you choose to take a year out after Foundation Year 2 (FY2), applications to all training pathways are made towards the beginning of FY2, meaning that you essentially need to be primed and ready by the end of Foundation Year 1 (FY1). Therefore, it goes without saying that your time at medical school is incredibly useful for working on extra items for your curriculum vitae (CV), such as audits, publications and presentations. Realistically, for any competitive specialty, leaving everything until you have graduated and are an FY1 doctor is not an option. Publications, for example, can have long periods from starting a project to eventual acceptance in a journal following review – it is not uncommon for this process to take more than a year. Therefore, a project started even during your first FY1 rotation may not be accepted (and therefore not be applicable to your CV) until after the selection process during FY2.

There are selection processes that occur even before FY2, further highlighting the need to start enhancing your portfolio as an undergraduate. Application for the Foundation Programme starts at the beginning of your final year of medical school and you are awarded points for publications, presentations and nationally recognised prizes as part of your application. This counts towards your ranking when it comes to Foundation school selection and the choice of jobs within this, and although this does not particularly determine your ultimate selection for later specialty training, getting the Foundation post you want is preferable. An alternative option at this stage is to apply for an Academic Foundation post. These will enable you to carry out research for a single rotation during FY2. These often provide you with teaching opportunities, depending on the programme, and are also a useful path to take if you are hoping to experience what life would be like as an academic clinician. In addition, the time spent doing research may result in a number of publications and presentations. Although these are unlikely to come to fruition ready for any selection processes you enter during FY2 (the academic rotation may even be scheduled after these), any achievements will undoubtedly be useful for any competitive stages at a later date. *See* Chapter 7, 'The academic training pathway', for more information.

ENTRANCE TO SPECIALTY TRAINING

Following your Foundation training years, there is a huge variety of career options ahead of you. You can make your first application during FY2, as described earlier. In general, there are two types of training programmes, dependent on specialty – run-through and uncoupled.

Run-through training programmes involve a single application at FY2 leading to a full training programme that culminates in your Certificate of Completion of Training, allowing you to apply for a consultancy post in the specialty. Progression from each year of training to the next is automatic, providing you satisfy all the competency requirements for each stage. Mainly used by the subspecialties, as well as general practice, it goes without saying that the single application during FY2 for these programmes is incredibly important, virtually confirming your career in the specialty to which you apply if you are successful and gain entry. This also makes many of these programmes incredibly competitive, and therefore you must ensure you are prepared for this early major step. At least considering how to enhance your CV while at medical school is highly advisable for application to any competitive run-through programme.

Uncoupled training programmes involve one application at FY2 to a common training scheme (usually 2 or 3 years in duration) after which another application is made to continue training in this field as a higher specialty trainee. As with applications in Foundation training, higher training applications occur in the final year of the Core Training Programme. For these applications you must ensure your CV is ready and you must prove that you have progressed from your original application made during FY2, demonstrating how vital it is to ensure you continue to enhance your CV during the intervening years.

Person specifications are available for the majority of specialties on the Modernising Medical Careers and deanery websites. Obtaining the person specification and any job application forms in advance can help you plan how to achieve, if not exceed, the stated requirements. Person specifications typically contain 'essential' and 'desired' criteria. Essential criteria are absolute requirements for consideration for such a post and must be fulfilled. The most important example of these are membership exams. For applications made during FY2, you are not expected to have passed any membership exams; however, for uncoupled programmes that utilise a second application to higher specialty training, completion of at least part of a membership examination is required for most applications. It is important to check the requirements for each specialty, as the criteria can be quite specific and this information is the key to ensuring you fulfil these requirements when it comes to your application.

A similar consideration of this nature concerns fellowship years abroad, which are commonly undertaken by higher specialist trainees near the end of their training. Taking such a post in the United States, for example, requires you to have passed the US membership examination equivalents before working there, so time out must be planned to revise for and sit an examination abroad before the anticipated fellowship year. As well as granting you access to working in the country in question, sitting extra examinations (in particular the US qualifications) are an additional way to boost your CV.

BEYOND APPLICATIONS TO SPECIALTY TRAINING

Stages of competitive application do not end once you have secured a place on your training post of choice. Applications need to be made for consultancy posts, staff grade positions and general practice posts (salaried or partner). In addition, the success of your career will be instrumental in making sure you are noticed when it comes to prestigious posts that are offered to the more senior and experienced clinician – managerial posts, professorships and even positions in the royal colleges. By the time of completing training, location will be a major influencing factor in job choice, as many clinicians will have started their own family, and staying competitive affords you a somewhat greater chance of being able to choose where you work. Alternatively, some may seek to work in particular environments (e.g. centres in which a super-specialised position is offered), and a similar tactic can help your application for these positions.

SUMMARY

Competitive applications are made at a number of stages of your career, knowledge of the pathway structure for your chosen career is absolutely vital, as well as knowing what is needed by which point. Ensure you work on your CV well in advance of each of these applications, as many things such as publications hold a considerable time lag and therefore careful planning is necessary to achieve the most by the time of application.

Section 2

How to plan for the future

Planning for the future, *your* future, is a very important thing to do, and the sooner you can do it the more it will pay off. This is not to say that if you do not start planning during medical school it is too late. Once you have an understanding of where you think you want your career to go, even in the loosest sense – such as paediatrics, regardless of whether you want to do paediatric oncology, paediatric surgery, paediatric gastroenterology or another of the many subspecialties – you are able to start focusing your portfolio and concentrating your efforts on this goal. As you move towards your preferred specialism, you will learn how to manipulate your focus to improve your portfolio for this new goal.

Understanding what you can do at different stages in your career will enable you to make the most of where you are now and it will also ensure you make the most of each stage of your career in the future.

This section will provide information on what you can do to optimise your productivity at each stage of your career, as well as giving you fresh ideas of how to approach aspects of your work that were previously thought to be mundane and a 'waste of time'. This will mean that not only do you engage more in your job and training, becoming a better student and doctor, but also you will be able to make more of your time and make sure that you are able to utilise your efforts to getting through the next application process.

CHAPTER 3

Medical students

Dr Nigel Mabvuure

INTRODUCTION

One of the fundamental differences between medical school and other university courses is that you are (almost) guaranteed a job at the end as a doctor. A medical student can therefore regard the first day of medical school as the first day of his or her career. However, this is only the first step in your career and it is where the guarantees stop. Specialties vary in their competitiveness, but even the least-competitive specialties located in sought-after locations such as London will be competitive. Most medical students have at least 7 years from the day they start medical school to when they have to decide on or apply to a particular specialty. This chapter offers some advice on what can be done in these 7 years to distinguish yourself from others and increase the chances of being admitted into a specialty of choice, in a location of choice. The first part considers academic achievements, as these are relevant to all medical students at all stages of training. The remainder of the chapter considers activities that can be done at various stages of training.

ACADEMIC WORK

It is likely that many of your classmates were towards the top of their high school classes. This can be a daunting thought for the student who wishes to excel academically. A more positive way of appraising this situation is realising that there is not that big a difference in academic potential between the top students and the bottom students in a medical school class. The differences in potential can usually be offset by the amount and quality of work one does. For the majority of students, it is more realistic to aim for accolades in a particular subject(s), perhaps those related to a specialty of interest. Remember that your future employers have been through medical school and are familiar with the calibre of medical students in general. It is probably more impressive to a surgeon that you were consistently a top performer in surgery and anatomy, but this is not crucial.

What impresses the most is consistency – you may find it easier to convince employers about your academic potential, regardless of particular strengths, if you have shown year after year that you perform to a certain standard.

Many medical schools award prizes for students who excel in particular subjects. Ensure you are aware of all prizes on offer at your school. Simple Internet searches will also reveal several national essay prizes open to all medical students. National prizes are more prestigious than local prizes and they also attract more points on job application forms. Unlike in the United States where all students take national examinations, these essays offer the only chance for UK students to assess their performance on a national scale. However, the calibre of these is usually high and they are only worth attempting where one has enough interest in the subject. It is also important to remember that the main reason for you to excel academically is to become a competent doctor.

RESEARCH

Research can be a rewarding experience for students but equally it can lead to disillusionment. The long summer holidays of the preclinical years provide an ideal period for interested students to begin their research careers. Many universities and national organisations offer summer research studentships by competitive application. Having well-laid-out plans and an appropriate supervisor increase the chances of success. Your medical school will most likely have a list of local and national funding opportunities but Internet searches may reveal more sources. At this stage you will not have much of a research record and the success of your application may lie with your supervisor's record. Look at researcher profiles on your university's website to note any grants these researchers may currently hold. The university's online repository and PubMed are useful tools to assess the research output of any potential supervisors. It may also help to choose researchers who have supervised summer students previously. The studentships can lead to publications and presentations but these should not be the main focus. It is more important at this stage to learn basic research skills, including lab techniques, statistics, referencing and scientific writing. The acquisition of these skills will also help future studentship applications.

The role of students in clinical research traditionally has been to collect data from patient medical records, tabulate it before presenting it to seniors who then proceed to analyse this and write up the results into a journal article or conference abstract. While this may be sufficient for students merely seeking to 'get their names on something', those interested in future research careers are encouraged to be involved in the whole process. There are numerous opportunities for clinical research in hospitals and this can usually be carried out alongside one's studies. Perhaps volunteering an hour a day to such projects may allow a good balance between course requisites and extracurricular research. There may also be funding available for these projects. Most specialties have national organisations, many of which encourage medical students to learn about them by offering grants for projects related to their specialty.

However, there are some pitfalls to research and publishing as a student. Ensure that issues of authorship and author rank are discussed with your supervisor early on. Many consultants will have projects they have wanted to do for a long time and they may suggest these to you. Do not accept a project on the spot but ask for at least two options; allow yourself time to read around the subjects before you make your decision. Also ensure that the bureaucratic aspects of research, such as ethics committee approval, have been completed. Although your supervisor may be responsible for the overall conduct of your project, you do not want your name to be associated with unethical work. Ensure that you do not commit academic 'crimes' such as plagiarism that may tarnish your research credibility for the rest of your career. For further information on research, *see* Chapter 13, 'R: research', Chapter 17, 'How to conduct research and publish your work', and Chapter 18, 'How to present your research'.

AUDIT AND QUALITY IMPROVEMENT PROJECTS

Audit and quality improvement (QI) projects involve assessing current clinical practice and identifying ways to improve it. Audits and QI projects can have a rapid impact on current practice, unlike research, which usually takes time before a sufficient volume of new research of a high-level evidence rating is accumulated. These types of studies usually do not require ethical approval so can often be started as soon as the projects are defined and planned. However, as these projects usually evaluate local practice, they may be difficult to publish in national or international journals. This should not put you off. They are relevant experiences that still attract points on application forms. To increase the chances of publication, audits and QI projects should have a generalisable message. Collaborating with colleagues in different parts of the country and repeating the same audit in each collaborator's respective location may achieve this. In this way, one can demonstrate national deficiencies in practice and these are usually of interest to journal editors, especially if solutions have also been suggested, tried and shown to improve prevailing practice.

PUBLISHING AND PRESENTING YOUR RESEARCH

The ultimate goal of research is to gain new knowledge and this is usually only worthwhile if disseminated by publication and/or presentation. Presentations and publications are a good way of demonstrating both the quality of your work and your commitment to a particular specialty. They also attract points on job application forms, making you more likely to be shortlisted for interview. Your consultant will usually not have time to write papers or may have many other projects under his or her supervision. It is up to you to draft research papers and send them to your supervisor for critical review and editing. Students should also note that original research articles are not the only way to publish articles. Many other opportunities exist, including letters to editors, commentaries on published articles and other formats specific to particular journals (*see* Chapter 13, 'R: research'). Most research projects require you to carry out a literature review prior to starting. It may be possible to publish these as narrative reviews that identify gaps in existing literature, hence stimulating new research. In selecting journals, it is important to select peer-reviewed journals listed on PubMed, as only these are awarded points on applications. Your supervisor will guide you with these matters and you should never submit any work until all named authors have given their approval of the final version.

Your work might be of a quality high enough to be accepted for presentation at a national or international meeting of a scientific or medical society. Oral presentations are more prestigious than poster presentations, but any presentation as a medical student is looked on favourably. There may also be medical student-specific prizes at these conferences, which are worth competing for as there generally will not be many students in attendance. Some societies also publish their abstracts in indexed journal supplements to attract more submissions to their conferences. There has also been a recent proliferation of conferences for medical students usually run by medical students. These can be rewarding experiences that provide good presentation experience in a less stressful setting. They also offer prizes and a few also publish their abstracts in journal supplements. However, these conferences do not attract points on current job application forms, although they are still relevant experiences to be seriously considered. For more information, *see* Chapter 18, 'How to present your research'.

INTERCALATED AND INTEGRATED DEGREES

Some universities require their students to take a year of additional study in a subject of the student's choosing. Other universities do not have this requirement for integrated degrees but offer their students the option to take an intercalated degree. Whether integrated or optionally intercalated, these degrees can significantly enhance a student's portfolio. There are several scholarships offered by national organisations to fund students with the best-laid-out plans and potential to succeed. These scholarships are extremely competitive but some students may begin to notice the benefits of accumulating the evidence of prior academic and research excellence. Unlike medical degrees, most of which are 'pass or fail', intercalated degrees are graded into classes depending on the level of achievement. For example, a student who gains a first-class degree can legitimately claim to have demonstrated high academic ability. The better your degree, the more points you gain on application forms. Intercalated and integrated degrees usually have a significant amount of time reserved for research. This allows students to carry out more extensive research projects, increasing the chance for presentation and publication in high-impact-factor journals. Remember that if you wish to be an academic doctor or to join a very competitive specialty, your intercalated degree may be required just for you to be competitive.

Since the rise in tuition fees to around £9000, the financial burden of intercalated degrees has significantly increased. Students not interested in being involved in research in their careers need to seriously weigh up both the benefits and the drawbacks of intercalating. The value of intercalated degrees beyond Foundation training is unclear and those who have not undertaken them can take postgraduate courses.

ELECTIVES

Electives are usually a much-anticipated component of the medical degree. Students have the opportunity to work in clinical and/or research fields of their choosing, usually in countries of their choosing. Students who wish to make the most of their electives should plan well in advance. The first decisions to be made are where to go and in which specialty to do your elective. The person specifications for registrar positions list elective experience as part of accepted evidence of commitment to a specialty. Students who know what specialty they wish to pursue are encouraged to seek opportunities in that specialty. In some countries, contact may need to be made years in advance. For example, students interested in elective attachments at the plastic surgery department at Groote Schuur Hospital in South Africa are advised to apply 2 years in advance. As with research projects, one of the most important decisions surrounding your elective is your supervisor. The speed with which your potential supervisor responds to his or her email may be a good indicator of how good he or she will be. This is particularly important if you are going to a developing country.

Once you have planned your elective, you can now concentrate on gaining the most from it. This starts well before you depart. There are many bursaries, scholarships, grants and travelling fellowships open to medical students for the electives. These are prestigious, as they are usually by competitive application. This usually means that a few students with the best-thought-out and organised plans accumulate most of the funds. Your prior research and academic achievements may support your application but remember that the most important consideration is your elective plan. Ask your medical school about general elective funds and consult the websites of your specialty's royal college or subspecialty's professional association for further funds. Experience shows that students carrying out research overseas have a good chance of gaining funding, as publications and presentations resulting from this mention the funding organisation. However, funding bodies do not wish to be associated with unethical research. Providing evidence of ethical approval will impress them, as it shows that your project has received independent review. Upon your return, you can still gain from your elective by presenting your work at conferences. Some journals accept medical student elective reports. However, the chance of publication is increased if you identify lessons that can be generalised.

LEADERSHIP

As a doctor, at some point in your career you will become a leader, unwittingly or by design. It is of interest to your employer to know that you are aware of what this involves and that you have the capacity to develop the requisite skills. It is wise to start developing your leadership skills as a student. There are many ways in which this can be done, including leading student societies, sports societies or social societies and by assuming occupational leadership positions. If you have an idea for a student society that is not currently available, approach your medical student society, as they may fund your start-up. Experience leading a small society may work in your favour when campaigning for higher offices, perhaps in your medical student society committee. In turn, previous leadership experience may lead to national- or international-level leadership positions.

EXTRACURRICULAR ACTIVITIES

All work and no play makes Jack an unemployable, one-dimensional job applicant. Remember that your employers are looking to appoint a qualified individual with whom they can enjoy working. Also, the shortlisting stage at interviews is usually highly selective of impressive candidates. Therefore, it may take something apart from the usual academic feats to stand out. Some medical students competed at the London Olympics and this will undoubtedly stand them in good stead. While the average medical student will not soar to Olympian heights, it is important to show that you have interests outside of medicine. It becomes increasingly difficult to reserve time for extracurricular activities once clinical medicine starts. Because of this, extracurricular achievement, on top of academic achievement, is a good indicator of other skills such as time management.

SUMMARY

There are examples of UK medical students who have started journals from the ground up, while others have set up successful companies. This goes to show that it is possible to achieve these impressive feats: it is just up to you to decide how high you want to soar.

CHAPTER 4

Foundation year trainees

Dr Natalie Smith

BASICS: GETTING STARTED

As you start your Foundation training, do not get too engrossed by wanting to know what path you should take; it is important to learn the basic skills and competencies of being a 'good doctor'. For at least the first rotation, concentrate on 'learning the ropes' and understanding what it is that makes a competent, efficient and safe doctor – this is the core of what it is to be a good doctor.

The main skills that are required of a good Foundation doctor include:

- producing a daily updated list for the team
- leading the ward round
- requesting, checking, updating and acting on pathology results
- learning how to, and when best to, request radiological scans
- presenting summaries of patients on ward rounds
- attending lectures – grand rounds, morbidity and mortality, multi-disciplinary team (MDT) meetings.
- ensuring your prescribing is clear and correct
- learning how to respond to resuscitation calls and how to be an efficient team member at these.

However, one of the most important things a Foundation doctor can do is enjoy the experience. There will be highs and there will be lows, this is not debatable, but these experiences will, on reflection, be part of the best 2 years of your life. This is most probably the first time you will have had so much time and money and you will make many friends, so make the most of it.

By mastering these skills you are more likely to be looked on favourably by your consultants (who write your references and assess your capabilities at the end of each rotation) and all other team members with whom you have to work on a daily basis.

DEVELOPING YOUR APPLICATION

There are basic areas that you need to address in order to put yourself into good stead for further training. Each of these areas can be tailored more specifically to your desired specialty when you are ready but, as a Foundation doctor, getting one audit with a completed loop on one rotation will look better than two unfinished audits, where the cycle has not been completed, in your preferred discipline.

The main areas of your portfolio that you want to consider when you are thinking about your future applications are outlined in the following list. Each of these areas scores points for the majority of applications, so focusing on these will ensure you are able to get the most out of your efforts.

- E-portfolio:
  - › reflective practice
  - › team assessment of behaviour (TAB), aka multi-source feedback
  - › supervised learning events (SLEs)
- Courses
- Audits
- CV and presentations (*see* Chapters 8 and 9).
- Teaching:
  - › informal teaching
  - › formal teaching
  - › teaching courses
  - › instructor
- Qualifications
- Continuing professional development (CPD)
- Management and leadership
- Information technology skills
- Commitment to specialty

E-PORTFOLIO

At interviews, the order of the interviewer's interests will reflect the order of importance to the application. This will involve investigating those things that are not the 'minimum' requirements – everyone has to complete the Foundation year competencies, so you have to consider why interviewers would spend lots of time asking about them, as they will not reveal anything new about the candidate. Therefore, the interviewer will want to find out about the applicant across the table and what sets that applicant apart from the others – what makes him or her unique.

Reflective practice

The most important advice for reflective practice is to do it as you go along. If you make a mistake, document it, learn from it and change your practice. This looks positive on your application. Everyone is human and makes mistakes, but it is how you adapt your practice in order to prevent similar errors in the future that is important.

There will inevitably be an interview station or an application question on reflective practice that is marked highly. A common example is: '*Could you please share with us a point in your career where you have made a mistake that has resulted in potential harm to patient care.*' If you do not have anything to say, you will find an awkward silence! However, do not fall into the common trap of trying to create a 'positive negative' – that is, saying something like 'I care too much' because you think this 'negative' will actually be seen as a 'positive'.

Be honest, be frank and say how you improve with every mistake, however small. The people interviewing you are invariably consultants; they will be in charge of your training and they will also be responsible for your actions. If you learn from mistakes, they will be happy knowing that any mistake will only happen once; if they are not happy with your responses, or if they think you are using a 'positive negative' to try to score more points, they may very well be thinking, 'I am not sure I want this applicant as my trainee, as it may come back on me.'

Team assessment of behaviour, aka multi-source feedback

In a profession in which team working is integral to good outcomes and can ultimately be the difference between life and death, how you interact with your team and how your colleagues perceive you are crucial aspects of self-understanding. Do not just request the minimum of 12 forms for the TAB, get as many as you physically can and learn from the responses you get. To simply pass the TAB you need to ask a variety of people, but if you want to improve your ability to understand both how other team members perceive you and how you can improve your team-working capabilities, it is important to ask as wide a variety of people as possible.

For example:
- doctors – FY1 through to consultants
- nursing staff
- ward clerks/receptionists (they have the best idea of your organisational skills)
- physiotherapists/dieticians
- radiologists.

What to do if you receive negative feedback ...

If you receive negative feedback do not worry, but do not brush it under the carpet either! It may be a positive event in disguise, as you do not always know how good or how poor your interpersonal skills are. Make sure you 'reflect' on any negative comments and make a change. Do not go around the hospital trying to find out who the culprit was, as your team will be writing the feedback with two things in mind: you and your patients.

Remember to print out your TAB summaries and highlight positive comments.

Supervised learning events

SLEs are the means by which you are able to assess your performance as a doctor. The majority of the assessments you undertake as a Foundation year doctor are SLEs. These can take many different guises, outlined as follows.

- **Mini-clinical examination**: this is assessment of individual parts of your clinical abilities. Assessments can be as focused, such as 'Examination of the cardiovascular system', where the process is relatively fixed, or they can be slightly more free, such as 'taking a history of a confused patient'. Having each individual area of your clinical skills assessed can highlight small weaknesses that get missed during the broader case-based discussion.
- **Case-based discussion**: this assessment is more 'holistic' than the mini-clinical examination. Here you usually choose a case (or have one chosen for you) that you have had exposure to on multiple occasions. This forms the basis of the discussion – *What made you think of this diagnosis? What makes you think of the differentials? How would you or how did you manage this patient? What would you do differently?* The discussion then usually moves on to the subject matter around the diagnosis. For example, in a patient with an ST-elevation myocardial infarction (STEMI), *what are the differences between unstable angina, a STEMI and a non-STEMI in terms of management?*
- **Direct observation of practical skills (DOPS)**: this is exactly what it says it is. You perform a procedure – for example, a lumbar puncture – and someone watches you and assesses your ability to perform this task. Once the person is happy you are able to perform the procedure competently and safely, he or she will 'sign you off' through a DOPS, stating whether or not you are safe to undertake the procedure on your own and unsupervised.

COURSES

Courses are vital if you want to show that you are more motivated and are trained to a higher level, and thus you are a more useful member of the team, than the other Foundation year doctors applying for the same job. Again, everyone will have the basic courses such as Advanced Life Support, as this is a core competency for Foundation training, but if you are able to get one or two more courses that benefit you and your patients, you will appear as a candidate who not only appreciates his or her limitations but also acts to address them. *See* Chapter 16, 'T: training', for further information.

Examples of courses include:

- Advanced Life Support – essential for core training applications and could be a discussion station at interview
- Advanced Trauma Life Support – do this if applying for surgery, anaesthetics, or accident and emergency
- Paediatric Life Support – not essential, but looks positive if applying for paediatrics or anaesthetics.

There are a plethora of courses available, with some being quite specialty specific – for example, a surgical skills course. This is a good point to mention when you are asked about specialty training applications.

AUDITS

An important task to have undertaken while working as a Foundation year doctor is an audit. Audits are the means by which hospitals assess whether they are maintaining the correct levels of patient care and, if not, how to change their practice to improve patient outcomes. While audits are important tools for hospitals and departments, they are also vital to you in many ways: they show you are able to critically appraise performance, a task that is crucial to any good doctor; you are able to spend time creating solutions to problems and you are not simply 'a cog in the machine'; and you are able to re-evaluate and identify which, if any, of your ideas have effected positive change for patient care. There are invariably points available for audits when you apply for a job, and the top points for interviews come for those who have an audit with the following four aspects.

1. *A completed audit loop*: you have done one audit, suggested changes for the department, and then re-audited to see if these have had any effect.
2. *You as named audit lead*: this shows you have done the majority of the work and have not just acted as a data collector.
3. *Published new guidelines or implemented a change*: this shows that your ideas for change are not simply 'tell nurses to undertake observations more accurately', but rather are collated to produce a new guideline or procedural standard.
4. *Poster presentation or oral presentation (local, national or international)*: this shows that not only is your work useful to your department but also you have thought about how this could benefit other departments in the country, and thus improve patient care in hospitals in which you have never even been.

As with a lot of medicine, producing quantity over quality is not a good thing. It is better to have one completed audit loop that has produced a new guideline, has been published and in which you are named as the audit lead than to have numerous non-looped audits that have simply had 'educate staff' as the improvement message.

It will be preferable to do an audit in an area of your prospective future specialty. However, this is not essential, as most people complete audits related to their rotations in their FY1 year.

The majority of hospitals run a Foundation Programme audit as a mandatory component for completion of FY1 – an example is 'Changing Practice' at Poole District Hospital. This is a good opportunity to be involved in an audit and there are often grants available to the top project, which subsidises you to give an international or national presentation!

If you can tie in patient safety with your audit, this will be a bonus! Look out for patient safety conferences where you can also present your work. More information on audits can be found in Chapter 12, 'A: audit'.

TEACHING

Informal teaching

Bedside teaching or ward round tuition to medical students is an ideal time to share your knowledge and practise your teaching skills; however, almost all people applying for jobs are well versed in this form of teaching. In fact, the majority of good candidates will begin their answer to a teaching-related interview question with something along the lines of: *'As well as the numerous informal teaching sessions and opportunities that I have undertaken as a part of my day-to-day work, I have also ….'* This shows that they are always thinking about teaching in their daily routine and that they are aware of how important this is to everyday medicine and improving the quality of the next crop of doctors.

Formal teaching

The majority of hospitals hosting Foundation trainees will also have medical students. This gives you the opportunity to undertake teaching and develop your teaching skills on a relatively tame and enthusiastic audience. If this is the case, ensure you take part in the teaching programme for students, and if there is no programme running at present, offer to organise this.

In your FY2 you can then get an approved allocated session on your Foundation Programme teaching course if you speak to your head of training; however, this may be better if you pair up with a registrar.

Teaching scores a great number of points on applications, but only for formal teaching. The points scored are lowest for those who just partake in the odd teaching session, they increase for those organising local courses and they are highest for those who are members of the faculty on a teaching course.

Feedback is essential for teaching; this is your means of finding out what the students thought of both what you taught and how you taught it. This insight is vital to improving your performance as a teacher, ensuring that the content of your teaching becomes more suitable to the audience and your actual ability to deliver the material improves. Give out feedback forms at all teaching sessions and use these for reflection.

Teaching courses

There are often teaching courses organised by each deanery. These are specifically aimed at doctors in training posts who want to begin to learn about how to effectively teach across a wide range of situations.

Instructor

There are multiple opportunities to become trained as an instructor in various initiatives. An example is the British Heart Foundation's Heartstart programme,[1] where people in the community are taught about the importance of, and techniques to perform, effective cardiopulmonary resuscitation. It is possible to join your local Heartstart organisation and undergo the training course to become an instructor. This can be extremely helpful in a number of ways: it will build confidence in public speaking, explaining medical conditions in lay terms, repeatedly reviewing basic life support and sharing knowledge with others.

For more information on teaching, *see* Chapter 15, 'E: education'.

QUALIFICATIONS

Extra qualifications are usually attained either before you graduate, in the form of an intercalated degree, or after Foundation training when you undertake a course in your eventual specialty. If you have a bachelor's degree this is fantastic, as not only will it provide extra points for applications but also it will have given you an experience that most others will not have had.

There are a few part-time, distance learning, master's-level courses that are aimed towards Foundation doctors. An example is the Master of Science (MSc) in Surgical Sciences offered by the University of Edinburgh in conjunction with the Royal College of Surgeons of Edinburgh (www.essq.rcsed.ac.uk), which is aimed not only at providing a master's level of education and assessment but also at preparing the participants for their postgraduate surgical examinations.

If you do not have a degree by the end of Foundation training, do not despair, as this is the case for the majority of people and you can make up for the points elsewhere. For more information *see* Chapter 14, 'K: knowledge', and Chapter 16, 'T: training'.

CONTINUING PROFESSIONAL DEVELOPMENT

CPD relates to the studying you do in your own time to keep 'up to date' with clinical practice. It is something that becomes more important as you progress through your career, as you have a variety of teaching and education sessions timetabled into Foundation programmes. However, if you start early, it shows further commitment to your specialty and also that you appreciate how important it is that you keep up to date with your clinical knowledge and skills. Therefore, if you keep a CPD diary from your Foundation years, you will have plenty of evidence to back up any statement where you say you know how important this is.

What can you put in your CPD diary?
- Teaching sessions you have attended
- Hospital grand round meetings
- E-learning modules completed (and you can reflect on these!!)

MANAGEMENT AND LEADERSHIP

Management and leadership is not something most people associate with Foundation year doctors, yet this is a vital skill if you wish to progress through the career pathway and perform well at each level. There are many aspects of leadership with which you can get involved around your hospital at a Foundation year level.

For example:

- mess president
- mess treasurer/events organiser
- rota coordinator (although these are mainly done through clerical staff)
- teaching programme director.

Outside of medicine (dare I say it! But yes, it counts), do you belong to a rugby club, a netball club or even an extreme ironing club (yes, one does exist …)? Are you a tour leader, a captain or a treasurer for your team or club? All of these are fine examples of leadership and management experience and they also contribute to showing that you are not a medical robot but rather human, with interests outside of medicine. More information on management and leadership is discussed in Chapter 11, 'M: management'.

INFORMATION TECHNOLOGY SKILLS

Yes, information technology skills score points too. Basic competence with Microsoft Office is sufficient, but if you have experience with computer programming or you have made your own app, mention it. If you are well versed with statistical packages, this is very useful for any research project, so again, mention this in your CV and application.

COMMITMENT TO SPECIALTY

Many specialties want you to demonstrate that you have not simply decided on that career on a whim but rather, you have considered this choice carefully and have suitable experience with which to base your decision. A great way to do this is to undertake a taster day or week within a specialty you are seriously considering.

When you organise this, try to make sure you personally meet the lead of core training for the specialty. He or she may even be at your interview! Other ways of showing commitment to a specialty include:

- attending the career open day
- reading the specialty-equivalent monthly journal – remember one or two articles you have read so you can discuss them if asked
- attending royal college events – look on their website, they will have a calendar full!
- keeping a logbook: surgery, anaesthetics, and accident and emergency.

SUMMARY

Last of all, here are a few tips (and yes, these have all been done before!).

- Do not miss the deadline for your application – these are not negotiable.
- Do not lose your certificates and paperwork – buy a sturdy folder and keep *everything* in there!
- Do not turn up late or dress inappropriately for your interview.
- Do not leave any of this to the last minute – a well-spaced and ordered progression of your portfolio speaks volumes about your motivation, organisation and the likelihood that when you say you enjoy these things, that it is the truth and that you have not done them merely to get a job.

REFERENCE

1. British Heart Foundation. *Heartstart*. Available at: www.bhf.org.uk/heart-health/how-we-help/training/heartstart.aspx (accessed 10 May 2014).

CHAPTER 5

Core and run-through trainees

Mr Michael Ghosh-Dastidar
and Mr Mark Cookson

Applying to enter core and run-through training is the first part of specialisation and it is of benefit to you to give this decision plenty of thought. Remember that the majority of training positions are currently advertised in November/ December of your FY2 and so your preparation and research should begin well in advance of this. When deciding on your career, you must consider a variety of things, from duration of training, competition ratios, eligibility criteria and quality of life, to the future and the changing shape of the National Health Service (NHS).

Only a few specialties currently have run-through training from ST1 onwards, and so the majority of junior doctors progressing from Foundation years will enter core training. If you do secure run-through training, you cannot simply sit back and relax. It is vital that you demonstrate continual professional development, as you will face competition points for subspecialisation at ST3 or later.

This chapter, therefore, is aimed at those first years of core and run-through training and how to maximise your chances of securing the career pathway or ST3 position you want. In particular, it will focus on improving your chances at being shortlisted in your chosen specialty.

The structure of core and run-through training has been discussed in previous chapters. This chapter is split into sections focusing on career choice and the important components of the person specification for different specialties. In order to avoid overlap with other chapters in this book, only particularly pertinent points will be mentioned.

CAREER CHOICE AND SHAPE OF THE NATIONAL HEALTH SERVICE IN THE FUTURE

The NHS and division of the workforce are changing all the time. Over the coming years there will be a shift of services towards primary care, as more general practitioners (GPs) take on the management of chronic diseases and newer roles such as healthcare commissioning. As a result, there will be an expansion in the required number of GPs. Currently, approximately 30% of junior doctors progress into general practice, but this figure is expected to rise to more that 50% because of increased need and a reduction in the number of placements in hospital-based specialties. Public health medicine is a specialty that is also expanding, as is psychiatry, where there are more training opportunities than trainees at present.

Conversely, some hospital-based specialties, particularly the surgical specialties, are shrinking and there are likely to be fewer training opportunities. Increasing subspecialisation, centralisation of certain surgical services, and improved medical or interventional therapies are reducing the need for patients to go under the knife. Surgical specialties are already oversubscribed, with high competition ratios, and many people do not get training jobs.

Within the practice of medicine there are more than 60 specialties, so do your research and consider personal, present and future factors when choosing your career.

PERSON SPECIFICATION

The importance of thoroughly reading and understanding the person specification for the specialty and level for which you will be applying cannot be stressed enough. Read this well in advance, not at the last minute, because its contents will guide you through preparing your portfolios, the application process and the interview stage.

If you browse the person specifications for different specialties at ST3 level you will see that they all share a common format, with 'essential' and 'desirable' criteria that candidates must demonstrate. These are grouped into the same core categories for all specialties, with slight variation of the contents.

Qualifications

During the first years of core and run-through training, many of you will have to sit exams in order to progress into ST3 or ST4. This is true for all surgical and the majority of medical specialties. In some specialties these are not essential, such as public health medicine and histopathology, and in others they are desirable but not essential, such as sport and exercise medicine. Where qualifications are essential, if you do not have them you will not progress, even if you are in run-through training.

Where qualifications are desirable but not essential, rest assured that there will be points allocated for the attainment of those qualifications when it comes to shortlisting. In the case of postgraduate diplomas and membership exams, we would strongly recommend that you sit these in order to improve your chances – for example, the Membership of the Royal Colleges of Physicians of the United Kingdom, MRCP(UK), before applying to ST3 sports and exercise medicine.

Higher degrees and academic qualifications are slightly different and these will be discussed later (*see* Chapter 7, 'The academic training pathway'). Remember that a number of specialties also have 'exit' exams for you to complete during your higher training.

Increasingly, an intercalated Bachelor of Science (BSc) is a desirable qualification to have. Generally, it is irrelevant which subject you choose and also whether it is a library- or a laboratory-based project. However, if you choose a laboratory-based project you will have more opportunity to publish and present work. Regardless, if you do choose to undertake a BSc then you should aim to get as high a mark as possible, because it is only likely to carry any weight if you have attained second-class honours, upper division (2:1) or first-class honours (1st).

It is important to check the person specification to determine the qualifications you need and the time frame involved – for example, at the time of application for ST3 and by the time of interview. On the whole, these exams follow roughly the same format across specialties. There is a written component, which comprises multiple-choice questions and/or extended matching questions that test your knowledge, and a clinical component involving real patients or actors as well as simulators or models to test your skills. Visit the websites of the respective colleges to find out about the specific format, duration and fees for these exams. For tips on how to pass these exams first time, you must speak to your peers who have already sat them. They should be able to advise on the best books to study from and relevant courses, and they should be able to recall examples of questions and scenarios. Further information can be found in Chapter 14, 'K: knowledge'.

Eligibility and career progression

The next major categories within the person specification are 'eligibility' and 'career progression', which overlap. These concentrate on establishing your competencies and experience. Clearly it is essential that when applying for higher specialty training you can demonstrate, with relevant documents, your achievements of Foundation and core competencies. During your early training you must remain organised and vigilant in getting assessments (DOPS, clinical examinations, performance-based assessments, 360-degree appraisal, and so forth) and sign-offs.

Pay special attention to your learning agreements. Sit down with your educational supervisors for a discussion within the first couple of weeks of starting a post to ensure you agree upon realistic objectives for you to achieve within the duration of your post. During core training some of you may find that you rotate through specialties that might not be directly relevant to your future career aspirations. Instead of letting those few months pass by, you should try to find constructive ways to make the most of your placement that may benefit your future career – for example, sit your membership exams, do an audit, work on publications. It is important that you are constantly adding to your portfolio.

Completing assessments, learning agreements and appraisals is labour intensive for all involved, but it forms an essential component of your portfolio. If you don't get enough satisfactory assessments, in the worst case you may end up repeating years. This, of course, also applies to run-through trainees, who have to demonstrate satisfactory progress at their annual review of competence progression (ARCP).

Consider carefully your rotational posts during core training. See what rotations are available from different deaneries prior to applying for core or run-through training. Remember that if you plan to apply at ST3 for something highly specialised, then gaining experience during your core training might be difficult. For example, not all deaneries will offer placements in paediatric or cardiothoracic surgery, yet a minimum 6 months' experience is mandatory before applying to ST3. Similarly, in specialties such as dermatology, experience is desirable rather than essential, although it is likely that you will be significantly disadvantaged if you do not have any direct experience when applying at ST3. Some of you may have to undertake additional years of core training in order to get appropriate experience in such specialties.

Research

Research is increasingly desired for juniors who wish to progress into hospital-based specialties and it can occur in a variety of forms.

Historically, if you wanted to apply for a national training number in a very competitive specialty, such as plastic surgery, then it was almost a prerequisite to have a postgraduate research degree such as a Doctor of Medicine (MD) or a Doctor of Philosophy (PhD). With the advent of Modernising Medical Careers things have changed a little. For some specialties there are now clear academic pathways, and this is discussed more later (*see* Chapter 7). Those who wish to pursue clinical pathways do not have to do this, as it is not an essential criterion for applying for ST3.

However, these higher degrees are always impressive. They do appear in the ST3 person specification for most specialties, as a desirable criterion either in the research or the qualification section. Therefore, having one of these additional qualifications will certainly score you marks at shortlisting, particularly if the research degree is complete. They are also useful talking points at interviews, and they help to differentiate you from other candidates later in life when applying for consultant jobs. However, a higher degree should not be taken lightly, as it requires a huge commitment over a minimum of 3 years, and so only candidates who are fully motivated should apply. There is no right or wrong answer as to whether to undertake one. It really is up to you.

Whether or not you choose to undertake an academic degree, you still have to boost this section of your portfolio in other ways. Clinical research projects are useful and are also very interesting, as they seem to be more directly related to patient outcome. Indeed, many aspects of setting up a clinical research project can create an impressive section to your CV, from application for ethics approval, to successful grant applications, to presentation of your results and subsequent publications. These important processes and skills can help improve your applications, as some of them are mentioned in person specifications. *See* Chapter 13, 'R: research', for more information.

Audits

Audits are part of clinical governance and every clinician has to participate, regardless of grade. If you are a run-through trainee you will be expected to demonstrate involvement in clinical governance at your ARCP, and audits are also extremely important if you are applying to specialist training. It is very easy to involve yourself in audit from early on, even during medical school. Older clinicians generally do not want to be ploughing through spreadsheets of data, or phoning patients at home in their spare time. If you are an enthusiastic medical student, they will happily let you take this work on and also let you run the projects. They can also give you ideas and supervise your own projects.

Audits will be discussed in more detail in Chapter 12, but the most important thing to remember is that audits are of most value if you have completed the audit cycle and the recommendations from your audit are sustained in practice. The audit also has to be relatively recent to your application, and it helps if it is relevant to the specialty you are applying for. Audits also act as a bridge to other research activities, as these projects can be presented at meetings and can also be published.

Presentations and publications

Presentations and publications should form part of your portfolio when applying for higher training. The two, of course, go hand in hand because any work you try to publish could also be sent to a meeting as a presentation, and vice versa. When it comes to presentations, you will score the most marks if you have presented at an international meeting, but if not, national meetings are good. You should aim to be the first author on as many of these as possible. Remember that a poster presentation is still a presentation and can sometimes carry as much weight as oral presentations. *See* Chapter 18, 'How to present your research', for more information.

Publications are an important component of your portfolio. Again, being the first author is preferable, as is publication in peer-reviewed journals (with a high-impact factor). There is a spectrum of publications from pictures, to case reports to original articles, but all can count and some take a lot less time than others to do. You can never have too many of these (and the same goes for presentations), but on application forms there is usually only space for five or six of your best. You can start early as a medical student, when you have more time. If you are enthusiastic, more senior clinicians will always be happy to get you involved in current projects, and to oversee and suggest other research activities for you to do on your own. More information on research can be found in Chapter 17, 'How to conduct research and publish your work'.

Clinical skills

Development of adequate clinical skills is a key component in progression to specialist training. Obviously the skills you need to develop differ depending on which specialty you are applying for, and therefore you should read this section of the person specification closely. Evidence of your skill base comes from assessments, validated logbooks, educational contracts and references. The most important thing that you can demonstrate is that you have made adequate progress for the amount of time you have spent within the specialty. So, for example, if you have spent 2 years in medical specialties and have never performed a lumbar puncture or a chest drain, you will pale in comparison with the candidate who has done several of these procedures within 6 months.

Attending recognised courses is another way of validating your clinical skills, and for almost every specialty there are certain courses that are mandatory. The most important ones are mentioned in the person specification, but don't limit yourself to only these, as other relevant courses are useful and you should document such courses on application forms. Your clinical skills are assessed through a combination of the work-based assessments and clinical skills training days as well as during interviews.

Commitment to specialty

This is a rather vague phrase that incorporates several different things. It essentially refers to what you do over and above your everyday job to further yourself within your chosen specialty. This includes practically everything we have already discussed here, provided it is relevant to your future career. So, any research projects, degrees, publications, presentations and audits that are directly related to your specialty demonstrate commitment. Prizes (especially postgraduate ones), such as for essays or presentations, are particularly good and differentiate you from others, as many candidates leave this section blank on application forms.

Similarly, enhancing your education and exposure within your specialty demonstrates commitment. This can be in the form of advanced courses, attending educational meetings and conferences, becoming an affiliate or member of societies or colleges, and so forth. Also important are your referees. You must have at least one referee who you are confident will fully support your application, and who also is a recognised and respected person within your chosen specialty. If you plan to apply to a specialty with high competition ratios, it will be of benefit to you to meet as many senior people as you can within the region and nationally, so that you are able to begin to understand the current and potential future structures of the specialty, as well as giving you access to people performing the cutting-edge research and thereby enabling your understanding of the specialty to develop.

Other areas

The other important areas where you must show development during your training is as a teacher and as a leader. Teaching is vital, and your role is continually assessed throughout your career and on application forms. You must demonstrate that you have experience teaching both undergraduates and postgraduates in a variety of situations, from bedside teaching to lecturing. You can consolidate your teaching by volunteering to examine medical students during their objective structured clinical examinations (OSCEs), for which you usually receive a certificate and this looks good in your portfolios. Undertaking a recognised teaching course is recommended – this provides additional evidence. Finally, to really impress, and to give you an edge over your competition, you should try to become a faculty member for a recognised teaching programme. This demonstrates that not only are you a good teacher but also you are competent and responsible, you have leadership traits and you are dedicated to your specialty. This is covered in greater depth in Chapter 15, 'E: education'.

As your career develops you will take on roles of increasing responsibility, leadership and management, regardless of the specialty you are in. Deaneries and trainers are expecting trainees to prepare for these roles earlier and earlier, and good candidates will stand out. You should think about how your portfolio demonstrates you have these qualities. Try to take on certain roles that may help, such as being the rota organiser or starting up a teaching programme. Others may choose to do leadership and management courses or even undertake extracurricular diplomas or degrees.

It is to be hoped that by focusing your efforts on the areas we have highlighted in this chapter, you should improve your chances of successful application to the specialty you want and also progress through your training without too much bother. You must also reference what has been discussed in this chapter with advice from senior colleagues within individual specialties, as it is difficult to generalise for all.

CHAPTER 6

Specialty training and beyond

Dr Nerys Conway

INTRODUCTION

Once you 'graduate' from core or specialty training you become a specialty registrar. This training programme usually lasts for 4–5 years, depending on the career and training pathway you choose to take. The requirements for this period of training are very different to those already encountered. By this point, you will be in the specialty within which you will spend the majority, if not all, of the rest of your career. There are no further stages of training that need to be applied for, only your consultant post.

As a registrar, you will need to develop a completely different skill set as you move away from being a junior member of the team to, ultimately, being the person in charge of the team. For example, you will be responsible for patient welfare and clinical management as well as training and education of junior staff. These are core aspects of being a well-rounded consultant and the very skills that you are required to develop over your registrar training.

Core training prepares you to become the clinician who ensures that patient care on a day-to-day level is kept at its optimum standard. This includes situations out of hours, as you may be the registrar on call for the whole hospital, so it is vital that core training has provided you with the skill set for this challenge. During your registrar training, you have to develop both your knowledge and your practical skill set to the level of that of a consultant. The clinical skills are developed through a mixture of experience and training courses, but there are several ways in which you can focus your energy to developing both your ability and your portfolio to ensure you are suitable for a consultancy post.

MANAGEMENT AND LEADERSHIP

Developing your management and leadership skills is vital to becoming a consultant, and it is a skill that you will utilise on a day-to-day basis. It is important to appreciate the difference between management and leadership. Leadership involves implementing change in a specific area or within a team. It involves developing people within a team to achieve their maximum potential in order to deliver excellent results. Management is about directing those within a team with principles that are already in place.

You may have had some experience of this already in your days at university or as a junior doctor. For example, some of you may have been captain of a swimming team or the 'doctors' mess' president at a hospital. These experiences will help you to gain insight into the managerial and leadership role required of a registrar. As a registrar, this may initially involve organising the annual leave rota for the junior doctors, leading a project within the department or attending meetings with senior clinicians. As a registrar you will demonstrate on a daily basis your role as a leader – you may be running the crash team, leading the ward round or being first operator in theatre. For those interested in management and leadership there are several courses and degrees available in order to pursue this interest. This is covered in more depth in Chapter 11, 'M: management'.

AUDITS

During your core training, audit was an essential part of gaining your national training number. As a registrar, your role in audit takes a slightly different approach. It is important that you encourage the junior members of the team to participate in an audit cycle and encourage them to submit their work as an abstract or poster presentation. For this, they will need both your supervision and your previous experience with audit.

Many junior doctors view audit as a 'tick-box exercise', yet audit cycles that are completed well can implement change and have a real impact on a department. Most junior doctors work within departments for between 4 and 6 months, so when choosing your topic it is important to bear this in mind. Some juniors will be willing to continue working on the same audit project when they have left a department, but this may not be feasible if they have moved to a different area within a deanery or between Foundation and core training. Juniors will be more willing to complete an audit in something that they enjoy, so it is important to consider their career choices. You may have more than one or two juniors completing audit at the same time, so it is important that you use this experience to develop your own leadership and time management skills.

Within your own subject specialty (i.e. acute medicine, cardiothoracic surgery, and so forth) you must also look at your own individual learning needs with regard to audit. As registrars we tend to stay within the same department for much longer, usually up to 2 years, but sometimes more. Over this time period we need to determine if there is any audit in that timescale that could have a real impact on the department in order to provide a better service for patients. This is something we can discuss with our senior staff with the aim of presenting it at a national conference (i.e. the Society for Acute Medicine, the Society for Cardiothoracic Surgery, and so forth).

A major positive aspect of being a registrar managing the audits for a department is that you are able to conduct a group of audits within a related area, which can combine to produce a result that is greater than the sum of the individual audits and thereby can create a real change to the department. Further information can be found in Chapter 12, 'A: audit'.

TEACHING

By the time you become a registrar the vast majority of doctors have taught junior doctors, medical students or other healthcare professionals. As a registrar you will take on a different role with regard to teaching. For example, there are more opportunities to teach at a senior level. These may include becoming an associate tutor to the royal college to which you are attached, teaching on a PACES course or organising the teaching rota within your department. As a 'specialist' you will also be asked to deliver teaching to doctors in other specialties. These are all good opportunities to improve your own CV, as well as to help the junior members of your team gain some teaching experience. Some of you may already have established by now that teaching is something you wish to become involved with at a later stage of your career (i.e. via the academic training pathway and practising as an honorary consultant). The first few years as a registrar will allow you to develop this and 'make yourself known'. There are degrees for those interested in medical education – they include a diploma or master's in education, available at various universities. More on teaching can be found in Chapter 15, 'E: education'.

RESEARCH

Research is not for everyone and it is not essential for every medical career, but for some, research is a fundamental part of their training, interest and career development. Regardless of whether or not you choose to participate in a research project, every doctor should have a basic understanding of what research means. Research creates knowledge allowing new standards to be developed.

At this stage of your career you may have the opportunity to participate in research by completing an MD, a PhD or other degree. In this position it is important to appreciate the key features of research governance and apply them to your own project. In summary, you need to ensure you gain ethical approval from relevant bodies, seek appropriate funding and liaise with the relevant institution or university. *See* Chapter 13, 'R: research', for more information.

EDUCATION AND CONTINUING PROFESSIONAL DEVELOPMENT

In order to progress towards a consultant post and complete your Certificate of Completion of Training you need to complete your specialty certificate examination (previously known as the 'exit' exams), usually in the form of a written examination. This is usually attempted in your third to fourth year of registrar training (ST5–ST7). Once this is completed you can progress to being a consultant.

The e-portfolio enables the deanery to ensure that you are reaching the right targets every year for your specific grade (i.e. ST3 competencies are less specialist and less comprehensive than ST7 competencies). The e-portfolio assessments are the same as those in Foundation and core training. All registrars are also required to keep a logbook of conditions they see, procedures or operations performed, and so forth. Every year the deanery invites each registrar for an ARCP. This is usually a 30-minute interview whereby you demonstrate to the deanery (using the e-portfolio, logbook, publications, and so forth) that you have reached a competency that enables you to progress to the next stage of your training. Further information on training can be found in Chapter 16.

OFF DUTY

Over the next 4 or 5 years you will be faced with some tough challenges, decisions and lots of hard work! Because of this your 'spare time' becomes more important than ever. Make sure you continue to pursue your own interests and hobbies, meet up with friends and family and treat yourself occasionally. Being a well-rounded person helps you become a well-rounded doctor – so relax and enjoy yourself, because after all that hard work you deserve it!

CHAPTER 7

The academic training pathway

Dr Liam Gillespie and Dr Guy Mole

INTRODUCTION

In 2005, postgraduate medical training in the UK underwent a large-scale transformation with the implementation of Modernising Medical Careers. A number of changes were brought in, including the introduction of the Foundation Programme, with the intention of providing greater efficiency and transparency in postgraduate educational training.

At this time a lack of education opportunities in research were identified and it was recommended that training programmes should be provided that offered trainees the opportunity to gain skills in academic competencies such as laboratory techniques, clinical research, medical education or leadership. It was on the basis of this that an academic training pathway was introduced. This runs alongside the clinical training pathway so that at every level of conventional postgraduate training there is an academic equivalent. Trainees can move in and out of this programme at the various stages; however, it was conceived with the intention of trainees progressing through all of the stages, and having been on the academic programme at the previous stage will advantage an application.

The route created starts with the **Academic Foundation Programme**, followed by an **Academic Clinical Fellowship**, which is equivalent to core medical or surgical training. Instead of higher specialty training you can opt for an **Academic Clinical Lectureship**, which ultimately leads to roles such as senior lecturer, honorary consultant or professor. Information on the academic training programme can be found online (www.foundationprogramme.nhs. uk/pages/home).

WHY UNDERTAKE AN ACADEMIC CAREER?

The most important reason for choosing an academic programme is an interest in research and academia. Within this, however, the options are extensive;

all major medical and surgical specialties will have academic programmes somewhere in the country and so will general practice, epidemiology, medical education and leadership. The last two are areas that are growing rapidly, with programmes in medical education focusing more on the role of doctor as teacher, while those pertaining to leadership concentrate more on the role of doctor in management. The more traditional academic jobs will teach skills such as laboratory techniques and statistics, which are gaining less emphasis in undergraduate medical education.

The programme is very advantageous in applying for both academic and clinical jobs throughout your career. It provides skills that will be viewed as an asset by future employers and which are very difficult to acquire on top of working full-time. The programme is also designed with incorporated time, funding and help from experts to help you obtain some of the additional CV items described in other chapters, such as higher degrees, presentations, teaching and publications. It also implies to those doing the shortlisting, and to interview panels, a degree of academic excellence, as these programmes are very competitive.

As already described, the academic training route has many advantages but this does come at a price. Trainees are required to achieve all of the clinical competencies that other trainees are, but, because of the dedicated research time, this has to be done with less clinical contact. As a result, academic trainees have to be very proactive in gaining the most knowledge and skills possible from every clinical learning opportunity and they have to be more organised in arranging sufficient clinical assessments to complete the necessary portfolios.

GETTING AN ACADEMIC JOB

In the final year of medical school, when applying for Foundation jobs you can also opt to apply for the Academic Foundation Programme. It is important to note that this is *not instead of* the Foundation Programme, as your application will be entered for the Foundation Programme if it is not successful in gaining an academic job, and so in that sense there is nothing to lose by applying.

The process is competitive. For the largest unit of application in 2012, which included the medical schools of London, Brighton and Sussex, there were 745 applications for 120 jobs, a competition ratio of 6.21 applications per post. However, this headline figure can make it look more difficult than it is, as each candidate could apply for three units of application. The application form looks for achievements in the same broad categories that will be discussed in greater detail in later chapters of this book, including teaching, audit, leadership and research. Many candidates attempt to excel in one area, such as research; however, it is worth remembering that there will be a maximum score for each category and so it is more important to score well across the board than to ace one section and fall down because you have neglected other areas of your CV.

Interviews now tend to be in an OSCE style with several short interviews, with your overall score an amalgamation of the individual scores. Most units of application have a station on research that you have undertaken and general questions about research or audit techniques, such as the different sorts of trials or basic statistical tests. There is nearly always a clinical scenario that, from talking to academic trainees from around the country, is normally management of an emergency, as the assessors want to know that you are safe on the wards, especially as you will have less clinical time than other trainees. Other stations are a bit more hit-and-miss, but popular topics are ethical and medico-legal scenarios. A common question seems to be to discuss a recent paper you have read, so it is always worth having one or two prepared!

The question of when to start trying to get things on your CV for academic jobs is easy to answer: as soon as possible! Research often takes years to publish, and it will not count unless accepted by a journal with a PubMed ID number. Other aspects such as teaching or conferences can be done in the later years, but make sure you always have objective proof, such as a signed certificate from your medical school – for example, showing that you taught OSCE skills to the first-year medical students.

ACADEMIC FOUNDATION PROGRAMME

The Academic Foundation Programme is the academic training pathway offered to new medical school graduates. Like its purely clinical counterpart, it comprises 2 years: FY1 and FY2. There are a number of ways in which the academic component can be incorporated into the 2 years, but the two main ways are (1) via a dedicated 4-month academic block at some point during the 2 years or (2) by having dedicated time set aside each week to run alongside your clinical jobs. The manner in which your time is to be allocated is not usually your choice but is made clear at the time of application. During the time dedicated to your academic training you will usually be expected to undertake some form of research project, which provides an ideal opportunity to gain a publication.

The application process for both the Academic Foundation Programme and the Foundation Programme seems to change drastically every year, but the key thing is that it is never too early to start looking into how to apply, or to start undertaking projects that may help to make your application more competitive. Individual eligibility criteria for entry onto Academic Foundation Programmes vary, but all will expect successful applicants to demonstrate not only an interest and ability in research but also exceptional clinical skills, as trainees need to attain the same level of clinical achievement in less time. A further BSc is pretty much mandatory and the requirement is for a first-class or upper second-class degree. However, this is by no means the only achievement that will be taken into consideration; publications in peer-reviewed journals, posters and oral presentations at national conferences, research grants for independent research prizes and awards that are given at a national level will all contribute to being shortlisted for interview.

An advantage of being on the Academic Foundation Programme is that you will be affiliated to a teaching hospital. As a result, you will not change hospital between your FY1 and your FY2 and so it will easier to complete any projects that are ongoing. In addition, a teaching hospital will have more opportunity in terms of research, as well as exposure to medical students to enable you to start developing your teaching skills.

ACADEMIC CLINICAL FELLOWSHIP

Any doctor who successfully completes FY1 and FY2 is eligible to apply for an Academic Clinical Fellowship, so even if you don't complete an Academic Foundation Programme you still have a chance of undertaking an academic training programme at the next level. The main purpose of undertaking an Academic Clinical Fellowship is to allow core trainees the opportunity to prepare to undertake a higher research degree, while still providing sufficient clinical exposure to successfully complete core training. An Academic Clinical Fellowship lasts for up to 3 years (4 years in general practice) and is considered complete when the trainee gains an appointment onto a training fellowship to gain a PhD or an MD. During this time, a trainee spends around 75% of his or her time in regular clinical work, with 25% dedicated to the academic component. This time dedicated to the academic component is longer than in non-academic core training, meaning that there is less pressure on completing clinical competencies than during the Academic Foundation years.

Like all academic training programmes, entry onto the Academic Clinical Fellowship is highly competitive. Although undertaking an Academic Foundation Programme is by no means a prerequisite, successful applicants will be required to demonstrate that they have gained suitable experience in research during their Foundation years, through peer-reviewed journal articles and presentations, in addition to being able to demonstrate that they will be able to continue to achieve the necessary clinical competencies in the face of reduced clinical contact, especially when progressing to specialist training.

While on the Academic Clinical Fellowship, trainees will gain a master's degree in clinical research, in addition to developing a body of research on which they will base their applications for funding for a training fellowship.

ACADEMIC CLINICAL LECTURESHIP

Academic Clinical Lectureships are intended to comprise a portion of your higher specialty training. Those undertaking an Academic Clinical Lectureship are expected to have already gained a PhD or an MD prior to starting. They are typically of 4 years' duration and time divisions vary greatly with different institutions; the academic commitment varies from 20% to 50% of your 4-year tenure. During the Academic Clinical Lectureship you are expected to generate research income for the university in the form of successful grant applications, and this income allows you to explore research avenues of your choosing. In addition to research commitments you will also have both an undergraduate and a postgraduate teaching commitment. These posts involve significant management expertise, as you will be expected to employ and oversee the activities of a number of doctoral students.

PROFESSORSHIP

Ultimately the academic training route was designed to create a route to professor so as to perpetuate the crucial advances in medical knowledge and treatments. Although it seems like a long route, you will still be at the highest level for longer than medical school and all of your training to Certificate of Completion of Training (including a PhD) put together. Therefore, if you are interested in having research as a substantial part of your career then this is by no means the only route, but is the one with the most expert help, funding and time to develop the research skills required in order to be an academic medic.

SUMMARY

Academic training programmes offer a fantastic opportunity to develop a range of academic skills. These skills can themselves provide a highly stimulating career or they can add valuable expertise to a clinical career. The key thing to bear in mind at any stage is that, although commitment to research and research experience are required to undertake any of the programmes, the manner in which these skills and experience can be gained is not fixed, and not undertaking an academic programme at one level does in no way preclude you from undertaking one at a later stage in your training. The CV areas discussed in Section 3 of this book need to be developed in order to get onto an academic programme but once on the programme you will have help and time to further develop your CV, giving your applications an advantage for both academic and clinical jobs.

Academic medicine is a difficult but highly rewarding training route. If you are interested in research we advise starting as early as possible, as it will always be easier to move back to a purely clinical career, if you decide that it is not for you, than to gain the necessary research skills to perform effective research while working as a busy clinician.

Section 3

How to get ahead of the competition

There are many ways in which you can optimise your score in an application or the way you appear to those vetting the applicants for a job. There are multiple facets that are applicable to most applications in medicine and, as well as making your application better, these will all improve your work as a clinician and your ability to work as an effective team member. Understanding the differences between a CV, a portfolio and an application form are vital, as this allows you to prepare each optimally.

The medical CV is different to almost all other versions of the CV, and this will be discussed in detail, as will the medical portfolio. These chapters aim to educate you about the two most important aspects – content and structure – as well as other 'little tricks' that can help set you aside from the rest.

What do you have to do to get a training post? This is the ultimate question on everyone's lips as they approach an application. The answer is both simple and impossible to answer. It is not possible to give an individual breakdown of everything needed for every training post in every specialty. However, the fundamentals are the same for almost every specialty, and here we introduce the MARKET approach. This useful acronym will allow you to ensure you cover the core aspects of most applications – management roles, audit, research, knowledge, education and training courses.

This section will cover the ways in which you can show yourself in your best light as well as how to improve your portfolio, CV and application forms for jobs. It will provide useful advice on what you need to consider, with plenty of examples to ensure you cover all of the bases.

CHAPTER 8

The medical curriculum vitae

Dr Matthew Smith

People from all walks of life, applying for any job, are advised to create a CV. Having a well-thought-out CV is absolutely essential to progress in the medical profession, and you will be required to create one at some point, regardless of the specialty you enter, be it pathology, general practice, surgery or something else. No individual would even be considered for any medical position, from specialist training posts to consultancy jobs or partnerships, without having shown an interviewer his or her CV, such is their importance. Ultimately, the medical CV does not greatly vary from the CV made by people in other professions, in that it is a relevant précis of your career to date. Therefore, it is a vital document for quickly showing off all of your achievements. The only difference is found in the items that are important to include, which will be considered later in this chapter. At this point, it is important to note that the CV differs from the concept of a portfolio (discussed in the next chapter); however, both a proper CV and a portfolio should be developed simultaneously to ensure both are updated accurately.

As a succinct record of your every position, achievement and relevant period of experience from across your medical career, an up-to-date CV is invariably useful for your own benefit, so that you can stay abreast of everything you have done since starting medical school. For this reason, some people also refer to their 'CV' in a figurative sense, without actually meaning a physical document. These people use the term CV as a cumulative concept for the sum of things people have achieved in their career (e.g. publications, prizes), particularly if they feel they have achieved a lot and feel like broadcasting the fact. This can lead to discussion about CVs being an emotive and often contentious topic, and it is important not to let this make you feel disparaged ('CV envy'). No two CVs will ever be identical, and as long as you know what you need to achieve for your career goals, don't let another person's CV influence you. It could well be the case that they have quantified every tenuous thing they have ever done on paper, which could potentially be disadvantageous when asked about by an eagle-eyed interviewer. That said, it is important to always be vigilant as to whether things you have done, such as a regional meeting, might actually be a useful asset for your CV.

THE LONG AND THE SHORT CURRICULUM VITAE

There are two types of (physical) CV in practice: the long CV and the short CV. The long CV acts as a record for your own purposes to document everything that you have done. This, rarely, will be shown to outside parties, perhaps only in the future when you have a website advertising your private practice or your own page on a university website as an academic. Despite this, it is still a vital tool for organising your career mentally and your progression towards career goals. In the long CV, everything is on display in a succinct, ordered manner, and areas that might be lacking can be easily recognised. As you strive to do more things to boost your career chances, it will likely become immensely satisfying to see your CV expand as you make additions.

The short CV is primarily indicated for showing yourself off to others. Usually this will be in the context of an interview for a new position, such as a training or consultancy post. The CV provides a logical and standardised summary of all that you have achieved, and it could well provide some of the framework for the interview itself – such is the temptation for interviewers to discuss things that interest them, or that might impress them. Therefore it goes without saying that a well-constructed CV (and portfolio, similarly) can help you steer an interview towards discussing your achievements. Unfortunately, the opposite may also be true, and glaring falsifications or carelessly written entries may lead to negative consequences. It is vitally important to exercise the upmost care when constructing your CV, particularly a short CV destined for an interview room.

CONSTRUCTING THE CURRICULUM VITAE

When constructing a medical CV, a valid question is how far back to go? For certain, anything before medical school is unlikely to be relevant (unless you won an Olympic gold medal while in the sixth form). Including anything from this period, such as being a school prefect, will undoubtedly appear as if you are scraping the barrel to interviewers when applying for a position. It may also serve to dilute your more recent achievements and take attention away from these. The medical CV should cover just that, your medical career, and even including A-level results is not recommended. As you progress through your career, older achievements or positions of responsibility lose their relevance. For example, when applying for a consultant post 12 years after graduating from medical school, stating that you captained the med school hockey team is likely to go the same way as the school prefect example. Again it is about relevance; if you were president of the surgical society and you are going for a consultant surgeon post, this may not be of great benefit but, if you were applying for a core surgical training post, this would be very useful in demonstrating commitment to the specialty. The CV is dynamic throughout your career and must morph to reflect your progress. One point worth noting is that publications and presentations are timeless, and your first case report as a medical student can still be included at any point, so the value of these career-boosting factors cannot be underestimated. The exception to this is where an application might ask for 'three selected publications'; in this case you should choose only your greatest and best.

The order of your CV should follow a tidy format utilising subheadings to denote each section. There is no hard and fast rule for the order; however, it is generally a good idea to begin with education. Here you should first list your medical degree, and then any other degrees you might have, followed by any courses you have attended. Following this the order is up to you, but you should make sure you include (if applicable) presentations, publications, teaching experience, positions of responsibility, book contributions, conferences attended, prizes awarded, papers reviewed for journals and any events run by you. The inclusion of any extracurricular activities should depend on how recent they were and whether it is something that might make you stand out. Proficiency in foreign languages, recent qualifications (e.g. high-level music grades) or participation in regular sports teams can show that you possess all-round talent, without sounding pedantic.

A difficult decision when constructing a short CV is what should be left out – clearly not everything can be included. Short CVs usually are assumed to be two to three pages long, unless instruction is given otherwise. Some disciplines give different lengths depending on the level of training, with more room allocated to those further along their training, reflecting the increased content expected of these applicants. Generally, sections on education, publications, presentations and books (should you have been lucky enough) are important inclusions. For other sections, perhaps consider using an abridged format. For example, if you were applying for a specialty training post and you were previously chair of the British Medical Association's Junior Doctors Committee, adding this would be highly recommended. Adding below that you were captain of the football team would be a waste of space, unless you could find nothing else to fill the limited space. The bottom line when drafting a short CV is to be thoughtful of what you add; think of what you are using it for, and what the interview panel will be most impressed by from your vast collection of achievements.

The overall presentation of your CV is also important; however, some people can be tempted to go overboard, even adding decoration, such as Roman columns down each side of the document. This is obviously over the top; however, do ensure that your CV is in a clear, non-distracting font, that reasonable spacing is used and that wording is sized appropriately. It is vital that your CV is as accessible as possible – pleasure the interviewer's eyes, not strain them. A final point is to make sure everything is dated meticulously – in particular, courses and conferences.

SUMMARY

Your CV is a vital tool for advancing your medical career. It allows you to summarise the achievements of your medical career and serves to provide a mental shelf for defining your progress towards your desired career goals. Starting a CV early is highly advisable, and although it may not seem to contain much at first, you will quickly find it filling up – this can be a highly satisfying process.

CHAPTER 9

The portfolio

Dr Matthew Smith

Similar to a CV, the portfolio is an integral tool for advancing your medical career. Maintaining a thoughtful and up-to-date portfolio is now a definite requirement for success when applying for training posts or consultant jobs, and applicants attending interviews without a well-constructed and comprehensive portfolio will undoubtedly leave a negative impression on their interviewers. Portfolios are also required at your annual review, and so keeping your portfolio up to date as you undertake new roles or have new achievements will ensure you are prepared for this stressful time.

A portfolio, in the simplest terms, is your chance to present all of your achievements to interviewers considering you for a position. However, before elaborating further on the rationale of building a portfolio and how to go about this, it is helpful to first define what a portfolio is and how it differs from a CV (discussed in the previous chapter). Although both are similar in concept, in that they allow you to display the sum of your achievements, the portfolio differs in execution. While the CV is a structured list delineating everything you have done in a logical fashion, the portfolio allows you to present these things under your own terms in a fashion that you see fit. Ultimately this comprises evidence of all of your publications, presentations and other important features and allows you to display far more information than a single CV entry representing the same point. Each page is devoted to one facet that represents an achievement of yours, and can tell a story clearly and more personally to the interviewer. Having assembled a portfolio, it demonstrates that you have reflected thoughtfully on your career and presented this for consideration, rather than just turning up to an interview hoping to get round to discussing some of your achievements. A portfolio may well be the basis for discussion in an interview, so it affords you the ability to influence the interview towards you before it has even started.

Let's consider, for example, that you acted as secretary of the surgical society while at medical school. You could show advertising or programme material from events that you ran, as well as a letter from the society president thanking you for your role over the position tenure. Clearly this latter point shows that a degree of tenacity may be required when looking to collate items for your portfolio; the president might not automatically offer to make such letters, but you could politely suggest the idea to him or her and offer to write a collective letter from the committee in return. When it comes to interview time – say, for core surgical training – the interviewers will see when they browse your portfolio that you ran a careers event (advertising poster, event programme), surgical skills evenings (advertising material, event photographs) and a Surgery in Schools event (letter from the Royal College of Surgeons of England), topped off by a thankful letter from the president summarising your enthusiasm and organisational ability over the year. This clearly conveys volumes about your enthusiasm and interest in surgery, and that you are willing to do far more than the minimum. A one-line entry on your CV, while useful, may well be lost among your many other achievements, and it can be questioned as to whether the surgical society actually did anything that year; the portfolio proves this.

So we have now established that a portfolio is like a brochure for your medical career to date: all the best points are exemplified in a clear and visually pleasing manner so as to advertise and prove how good you really are. Now let us look at what you should include and how this should be presented.

PRESENTATION

When starting your portfolio, it is important to remember that presentation matters: it shows that you care about and take pride in what you have done. The basis for any portfolio should be a ring binder in which you can collate all of your portfolio items. It is definitely worth spending a bit of extra money on a good folder, one that is sturdy and looks professional. This latter point is vitally important: don't go for folders with bright colours or bold patterns. In general, plain colours such as black, white or blue are the best, and patterns should be subtle and kept to a minimum. Some folders can be bought that look particularly ornate, with fine detailing in the design; this is appropriate as long as it is not over the top. Remember that first impressions are vital, and the portfolio is your sole brochure. Start with a smart folder and the rest of the portfolio will appear to be a lot more impressive than if you use a moth-eaten, old folder – remember, first impressions last!

Within your portfolio, it is highly recommended that you use plastic wallets. This will ensure no items become damaged or ragged and will give a tidy, uniform look across all of the pages. They are also much easier to turn when an interviewer is viewing your portfolio. The happier and easier you make things for the interviewer, the better – it all counts. When using plastic wallets, a difficult question is whether to use both sides of the wallet, like a book, or to display a single item in each sleeve for emphasis. There is no right or wrong answer: if you have accrued a large portfolio it is probably wise to use both sides to save on space; likewise, using one side only can make your portfolio look larger if you don't have so much yet. Whichever you choose to use, do ensure that you maintain this consistently throughout the portfolio; failing to do so could lead to items being easily missed. For example, if the portfolio starts out single-sided and for some reason you place your randomised control trial published in the *Lancet* on the reverse of a page, it is likely to missed by interviewers. The portfolio is mostly about maximising the visibility of your best achievements.

Another important point in this vein is to make sure that each item gets its own wallet or side. Do not place things that you would want displayed behind something else in a wallet, even if it is similar in nature. The interviewers do not have time to physically take your portfolio apart; if you cannot see it then the interviewers are not going to notice it. The only possible exception to this is where you may have included feedback forms for a teaching event. Make sure the most flattering one is visible at the front, and place the others behind; the interviewers will not take them all out but they can see that you taught a number of people by virtue of the thickness of sheets in the wallet. Furthermore, it would be inappropriate to put 30 feedback forms from one teaching event in individual wallets; this would simply waste time in an interview and would very likely bore the examiners.

As well as presentation, the structure of your portfolio is of equal importance. Think of your portfolio as describing the narrative of your medical career; you want this to seem as tidy and ordered as possible. Make sure that the portfolio has defined sections containing each type of achievement and its evidence. The use of card or plastic dividers is essential to define the structure and to act as a reference to the interviewer, allowing him or her to jump to a particular section. The portfolio should begin with the basics, and it is recommended that you begin with your CV (this acts as a kind of contents page), your General Medical Council (GMC) certificate and then medical degree (assuming that you have these by this point – these can be copies, so long as they are of the highest quality). Following this, the structure should roughly follow the sections in your CV, but ensure that it is still logical: publications and presentations should be adjacent without having a section on teaching experience between the two.

One final point worth considering on the topic of presentation is the labelling of evidence. For example, placing a set of feedback forms from a teaching event may be definitive proof you provided teaching, but what this was may not be immediately obvious. Here it would be pertinent to place small stickers in the corner of the plastic wallet, with a sentence stating what the portfolio item represents, along with a date.

TYPES OF EVIDENCE

There are numerous types of evidence that can be used to represent your many achievements; the important concept to consider is the need to physically quantify everything that you have done. Here we will briefly consider appropriate portfolio items for the main things you should include in your portfolio. This is by no means exhaustive – everyone's experience is unique and you may be able to obtain something useful not stated here.

For your educational achievements, the best form of proof is certification.

Certificates from degrees are essential (e.g. BSc, PhD), and here you can also quantify any postgraduate courses you have attended by providing the certificate of completion. Certificates of any prizes can also be used to prove their award.

For presentations, nearly all conferences these days provide certificates of attendance, while a few provide certificates confirming that you have presented. While it may be possible to ask for the latter, it is important to take a high-quality photocopy of the abstract book page and display this alongside the conference certificate. If an abstract book proves to be elusive for whatever reason, a neat presentation of the acceptance email would just about suffice. Don't forget to also include certificates for conferences that you have attended but not presented at. For local meetings, keep copies of the meeting programme for your records.

Publications are most likely the simplest to quantify, by their very nature. It is probably only necessary to include a printout of the first page of the article with your name and the title, especially if the paper is many pages long, as this would quickly fill your portfolio at the expense of anything else. Audit certificates from your hospital are also great additions, even if you went on to publish the data from an audit; this demonstrates that you are cognisant of the audit cycle as well. If you have written any books or contributions to one, these can be demonstrated by a copy of the cover or the chapter header, and possibly by documentation of acceptance for publication.

Evidence of teaching experience is ideally given through the use of feedback forms; however, a letter confirming your activities from a supervisor would suffice in their absence – the inclusion of both would be preferable. If you ran a specific teaching event rather than teaching on the ward, including advertising material, event programmes and even photographs of the event is an ideal way of showing off what you organised to the interviewer. The same also applies to any other type of event that you organise – for example, a talk from an eminent speaker or even a social event (photos may be less appropriate here). Positions of responsibility, such as being the representative for your deanery, should be proven with a letter from your superiors.

Evidence of extracurricular achievements can be useful but should definitely be confined to the end of a portfolio. These are particularly appropriate if you are especially talented in your field (high-performing athlete or musician) or you take on a position of responsibility (e.g. teaching English as a foreign language in your spare time, on the committee of a reasonable university society in earlier years of your career). Proficiency in other languages is particularly useful, as is involvement with a medical school society. Involvement in large and highly relevant societies, such as a paediatric or a surgical society, may even warrant a section of its own, and this should be at the beginning of the extracurricular section. This kind of achievement can be quantified through certificates, event programmes and letters from superiors; here your imagination and some lateral thinking may be required, as this is where peoples' unique contributions are displayed.

SUMMARY

The portfolio is a vital tool to display your best credentials to interviewers and it should be deemed essential to anyone. Starting early (i.e. at medical school) is advisable, as it would be nigh on impossible to go back to ask for a letter about heading up a society or the like 5 years later. The most important thing to remember is that the portfolio provides the shop window for your medical career; you can dress it up as much as you want to give the very best impression and rightly demonstrate all your hard work to those who need to scrutinise it. Without going overboard, include everything and seek to quantify all that you do.

CHAPTER 10

Marketing yourself

When creating a portfolio there are several requirements that need to be met. First and most important of all, does your portfolio show that you are someone who meets the person specification? If you are unable to do this then you are unlikely to progress into the job you are applying for. Second, does your portfolio highlight all of your personal achievements? Third, does your portfolio cover all aspects of the MARKET assessment tool?

Most person specifications are broadly similar, but then many people have similar portfolios. Therefore, there is the need to improve your portfolio to make you 'stand out from the crowd'. An appreciation of the minutiae of the similarities and differences between different person specifications is beyond the scope of this book, but these can be found as a result of a simple online search using the terms '*XYZ person specification*', where XYZ is the specialty you are applying for.

Speaking to consultants is a great way of understanding the specialty, but in this ever-changing environment that is growing in competitiveness all of the time, it is necessary to understand exactly what it is that is expected of all job applicants, and this can only be achieved by investigating the person specification.

All people applying for a job will have a medical degree; the majority of people applying will have one or two other things that they think sets them apart. For example, intercalated degrees, while excellent, are starting to become the norm rather than the exception. Therefore, to set yourself apart from your fellow job applicants you need to show a little bit extra. It is quite obvious that the sooner you start to address these aspects of your portfolio, the more you will have to show when the time comes for a job interview.

It has been said many times, and cannot be said enough, that being average across the board is better than being excellent in one area and below average in all of the rest. Think about it. Would you prefer to employ someone who had one research paper published, one conference presentation under his or her belt, had done some formal teaching, had evidence of completing an audit, had taken some postgraduate qualifications and had undertaken a post in a management role; or would you prefer to employ someone who had six papers published and no evidence of teaching, management, audit, presentations or taking postgraduate qualifications? Reading this it becomes obvious. If you have a paper published and you are offered an audit or a paper, then the audit would make you look a more well-rounded candidate.

The following chapters in this section will discuss in further detail the MARKET approach – this stands for Management, Audit, Research, Knowledge, Education and Training (*see* Figure 10.1). This is a systematic approach to improving your portfolio, resulting in a well-rounded end product that should cover the majority of the person specification for the majority of jobs. There will of course be small areas where different person specifications require other evidence of work, but having a well-structured and well-rounded base will ensure that meeting the requirements is much easier.

M	Management	Leadership roles Society involvement Involvement with journal editorial teams
A	Audit	Complete audit cycles
R	Research	Research papers published in journals Conference presentations Conference posters
K	Knowledge	Postgraduate examinations (MRCP(UK), Diploma of the Royal College of Obstetricians and Gynaecologists, etc.) Other higher education qualifications: postgraduate certificate or postgraduate diploma, BSc, MSc, MD, PhD
E	Education	Formal teaching roles Anatomy demonstrating Clinical teacher at a medical school/postgraduate deanery
T	Training	Postgraduate training courses (e.g. Basic Surgical Skills course through the Royal College of Surgeons)

FIGURE 10.1 The MARKET system of portfolio appraisal and improvement, with examples of each

There are many ways of approaching your portfolio, and simultaneously making any application look more impressive, but utilising a combination of two distinct approaches covers everything you need to do and allows for the most efficient use of time. First, a planned approach to 'cover all the bases' means that you are able to create the well-rounded application that will make you appear an excellent candidate. Second, there is the 'opportunistic' approach. Everyone undertakes this to some extent; if offered a chance to be involved with a research project, most would say yes and would benefit from this. However, being proactive in this is something that will allow you to set yourself apart from the other applications for your dream job. Examples include asking to write a case report on a rare presentation to your hospital, offering to undertake an audit, or setting up a teaching programme at a district general hospital where students are on placement.

By being proactive, you are not waiting to be offered a project (which may never happen) and you are able to control your destiny to some extent – you cannot dictate who comes into hospital, but once you see this rare case, offering to write this as a case report will go a long way to helping your applications in future.

Through a combination of planned and opportunistic approaches, it is possible to optimise your portfolio while covering all bases. This requires a shift in mentality, whereby you try to see the opportunity in your everyday clinical practice. However, once you do this, you will soon see that opportunities abound in a hospital for an enterprising doctor who is motivated and driven enough to bring about a positive change to his or her portfolio.

CHAPTER 11

M: management

Management is the area of medicine that is concerned with how you lead teams and services, as well as how you interact with people from different departments to ensure the greatest outcome for all patients in a healthcare service. Many will know that consultants are team leaders, and the hospital chief executive is the person in charge of the running of the hospital. However, there are a multitude of management roles within each grade of healthcare professional, with many different members of each team being involved with certain aspects of the team's management.

Management can come in several guises, from being the person responsible for the running of a hospital to being the person charged with making sure that there is enough tea in the doctors' mess (a very important person indeed!). Throughout your career, while you will be able to apply for many different management roles, some are thrust upon you by your consultant.

Whatever the situation, management becomes increasingly important as you progress through your career, and it is vital when applying for consultancy posts. As with all things in medicine, if you show a long track record of successful performance in management roles from medical school and through every grade of your professional career, you will look much better and more genuine when you say, '*I find management roles rewarding*' in your interviews, than someone who enters into 10 different roles in their final 2 years of registrar training to 'tick the box'.

On that note, every aspect of management is not for everyone. Finding what *you* are best at will mean that you find the experience more rewarding and also that you give more to the people whom you are managing. If you are an extroverted, outgoing person, then teaching and lots of face-to-face work may be your best avenue, while if you are more introverted, you may find that you are more suited to running the departmental audits or organising the staff rota.

Simply doing management roles to tick a box on an application form may work at the lower ends of your career, but as you progress, it becomes more obvious if this is the case. Therefore, do not see a management role as something that has to be done to get a job; rather, see it as something that, if chosen carefully, can provide you with great enjoyment, is a learning experience and can also provide your patients with improved standards of care.

If there is no management role at your trust and you feel that there is something that can be done to both improve the efficiency of the hospital and improve the impact of the hospital on the surrounding community, there is nothing from stopping you from creating this post. This is more work but you will be sure that this is something that you want to do and you will also benefit from being able to mould the role into exactly what it is you think it should be. This also looks exceptional on any application that you submit, as it shows initiative, creative thinking and a level of critical thinking in your daily work. So, do not be put off by 'Sorry, that role doesn't exist'. Be persistent, speak to your consultant, your Foundation Programme manager, your deanery, the chief executive of the hospital, anyone who you think has the authority and power to be able to say, 'yes, let's do it!'.

The remainder of this chapter outlines possible roles broken down by career grade, from medical student to senior registrar, but this is by no means a list that is comprehensive. This will show you a diverse range of management roles and also provide you with ideas to create your own roles if they do not exist in your current training post.

MEDICAL STUDENTS

It is very easy to become a medical student and think, 'Great, only 5 years and I am a doctor'. This is true, barring a few examinations on the way, but the vast majority of people pass medical school exams, and if you apply yourself, you will certainly do so. However, every single doctor in the world has a medical degree. While this is an amazing feat, it is by no means your golden ticket to your dream job. Management roles are plentiful at medical school, and to make them even more enticing, there is usually something available in your hobby, so you can combine your interests with making yourself look better for the future, as well as making the medical school experience better for a lot of other students.

The most obvious positions are those of 'MedSoc', or the medical society of your medical school. Here you will be an integral part of the cogs of student life. There are roles as diverse as president (the big cheese and in overall charge), social secretaries (for those who enjoy socialising) and treasurer, and many, many more. There are also year representatives, where you can champion the causes that are close to the hearts of your fellow year members.

Other than MedSoc roles, which some people find too grand and not focused enough, there are the individual societies. These are what make a medical school hum with excitement, interest and action. You can become a member of a current society or start your own. They range from sports to academia and the arts. There is literally nothing you cannot create a society for if there is an interest at your medical school. Within each society are similar roles to those of the MedSoc roles – president, vice-president, treasurer, secretary, social secretary and year representatives. If there is no existing society, if you have a motivated group of students, you can form your own society, but be aware, this is a little more work than simply becoming president of an existing society, although it is also more rewarding.

Most medical schools have student representatives who sit on a multitude of panels and boards, where decisions are made about the general direction the medical school wants to take in the future. These meetings welcome student input, as the students are the ones who will have to live with the consequences of these meetings.

Outside of your medical school, there are plenty of different roles available to you. The Royal Society of Medicine (RSM) has many different 'sections' (e.g. the psychiatry section) covering almost all aspects of the medical profession, and each section has a student representative. Here you can work closely with senior consultants, giving you an understanding of what it is that is required to run such a committee. There is also the Medical Students Committee at the RSM, which has up to four representatives from each medical school and is tasked with facilitating the link between the interests of the postgraduate arm and those of the medical students.

Other than this there are representatives for medical students at almost every different postgraduate college. These are fantastic ways of not only boosting your CV (which should be seen as a bonus point and not the motivating factor) but also meeting like-minded people, exploring all that these specialties have to offer, and identifying if you think you connect with that particular branch of medicine.

One cautionary note: do not take on more than you can manage. Medical school is a roller coaster of commitment, with several deadlines usually coinciding in a short space of time. There is nothing worse than not being able to deliver on promises because of your other commitments. It is better to undertake one or two roles during your time at medical school and maximise your experiences and learning from them than to take on lots of roles but at a very superficial level.

FOUNDATION DOCTORS

It is very simple to think 'I have made it' after graduating. It is perfectly normal to think that you have arrived on the career escalator and, in no time at all, you will be sitting in the consultancy interview extolling your virtues. However, Foundation training is unmatched in its potential for you to demonstrate who you are and who you want to be professionally. There are as many roles available to Foundation doctors as there are to medical students, but you can now extend your focus to national and international roles.

Foundation deaneries have various roles within them for trainee representatives, much in the same way medical schools do, but these are usually spread across the whole deanery and as such are slightly more competitive, although there are usually enough roles to go around. Again, if there is not a role that you think should be there, then why not propose it to the deanery?

Once you are in Foundation training, you can start to get an idea of the general specialty in which you wish to spend the rest of your professional life (anaesthetics, surgery, general practice, medicine, and so forth). If you have made this decision, then it is possible for you to become more actively involved with societies within these specialties. Most of these groups tend to offer medical student membership, but not all have positions for medical students on the faculty. This means Foundation trainees can become members and really make a difference, as they can represent the views of medical students and Foundation doctors while also gaining further experience in how to work as a representative, how to undertake roles within a society and how to work with many different people to reach a common goal.

CORE AND SPECIALTY TRAINEES

Core trainees have usually nailed their colours to the mast. They are usually in the system for a specific general specialty, be this general practice, general medicine, general surgery or one of the run-through programmes such as paediatrics. Once you have done this, it can be a lot simpler to make decisions regarding management roles. As with medical students and Foundation trainees, it is possible to become involved with societies, but it is now easier and more useful to start working within your chosen specialty; for example, if you are a core surgical trainee, becoming a faculty member of the Association of Surgeons in Training, and approaching individual sections of the RSM as well as applying to work with national societies to help organise a national or international conference in your specialty.

Other things that may be possible include becoming a team lead for different roles within the hospital. Here you can supervise the audits that your team produces, or you can organise the departmental journal club. These simple but often loathed jobs can provide excellent education in how to organise teams and ensure people keep to schedule, and they can also give you insight into how you work as a manager – are you very hands on? Are you able to delegate easily? Are you able to identify those who need extra help and those who can work independently? Learning the answers to these questions will ensure that you are better equipped to tackle these tasks in the future, and that you are able to address your personal skill shortcomings and start to improve your ability to be a team leader.

SPECIALTY REGISTRARS

So, you have made it this far. You are 'the Reg' – the person with a lot of responsibility and an even greater workload. At night, you will probably be the most senior person in the building in your specialty and people will turn to you in their moments of need. This role is, by definition, one of management; you are running teams, especially at night, and you are tasked with overseeing a lot of the routine work that your department does. However, simply saying 'as the registrar I was in a management role looking after my team' shows that you have done your registrar training but nothing out of the ordinary. This is the time when you can start to become the person on the ground who organises lots of other projects, the master puppeteer if you will. Here you can oversee the teaching, audits and research of the department; you can set the themes of what you want to happen, get those involved to work to an agreed plan, and manage the quality of what is produced so that everyone involved gains maximal benefit from their efforts. You are also able to become a member of a training course or conference faculty. Here your management is entirely different to that of anything else you will have experienced. Rather than organising people you work with daily, you will need to have a completely different communication pattern, as this is often a responsibility split over vast geographical distances, with the sole aim of bringing a course together in one place.

SUMMARY

Management is not all about sitting in an office: it can be running a society, it can be overseeing your department's audits, it can be almost anything. The limit to your management experience is your imagination. There is a management role for everyone, and it is not possible here to go into the detail of every single position available. In this chapter we have given you a brief overview of what management is, why it is important, and also some ideas of what you can be thinking about during your career. Management is something you have to demonstrate on your application, but it is so much more than that; if done properly and approached in the right way, it can teach you more about yourself and the subject matter than any training course. This is the real bonus of management: you are no longer just a cog in the machine, you are the controller of the machine and for that you have to appreciate what each cog is doing and that is one of the best educational experiences that you can have.

CHAPTER 12

A: audit

THE AUDIT PROCESS

An audit is a quality improvement process that seeks to improve patient care through the evaluation of procedures, departments or hospitals to a standard or guideline to see if they meet a minimum level of acceptable performance. The ultimate aim is to improve the quality of patient care and to ensure that best practice is being carried out and is in line with the latest evidence and guidance. If it is found that the level of care does not meet the minimum standard, changes are implemented to ensure improvement. If standards are above the minimum, it is still possible to improve practice, unless compliance is 100%.

Audits are crucial to clinical care and your personal education. Audits are the very heart of 'problem-based learning' and are essentially a formalised way of recording what it is you should be reflecting on after each patient you see. The questions are essentially as follows.

- *'Did this patient get the best possible care?'*
  - ❯ If so, repeat this process when faced with the same clinical situation. If the patient did not receive the best possible care then you need to be asking yourself why not and …
- *'What could I do better next time?'*
  - ❯ Here you investigate what it is that you should do to make the standard of care better for the patient next time you are faced with the same clinical scenario. Consider best practice recommendations and how your practice differed from this in order to evaluate how best to approach the same clinical scenario in the future. Once you have considered how to improve your practice then you can …
- Re-evaluate your performance.

This is how all doctors think with every situation and it is how we improve our performance, knowledge and patient care. An audit is basically a service-level improvement process.

The most important part of the audit is to 'complete the cycle'; that is, to re-audit the same parameters to see whether the changes implemented are being followed and allow the audit subject to meet the minimum standards originally set or even to improve above the minimum standards. Even if you move on to different places it is important to ensure that someone else completes the audit cycle. Without the re-audit it is impossible to know whether the changes implemented have been for the better (*see* Figure 12.1).

An audit is a simple and easy way to show that you have participated in research and it does not have to be big or complicated. It is a good idea to discuss doing an audit with your registrar or consultant, as he or she may be aware of ongoing audits with which you can get involved or may be able to give you some ideas of potential audits to start.

While audits can be easy and simple, it is still a good idea to do an audit in an area that interests you and not just for the sake of doing an audit. While any audit looks good on a CV, an audit in the area in which you are interested shows commitment to and interest in the specialty prior to interviews.

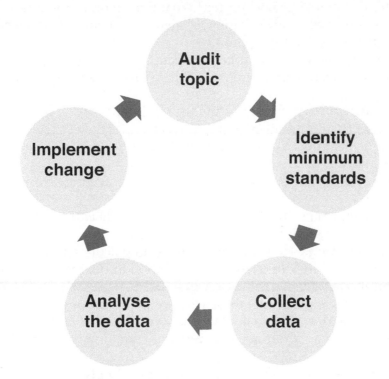

FIGURE 12.1 The audit cycle

PLANNING AN AUDIT

When planning an audit, it is crucial to consider various things to ensure your audit is investigating performance in an area that is important to service provision or patient care, that it is investigating what it aims to investigate, and that the methodology is sound so that the results are indicative of the clinical situation. The following steps should be considered.

- *Audit design*: Is the audit concerned with evidence-based medicine in practice (e.g. are patients being assessed for nutritional status using the malnutrition universal screening tool (MUST) score?) or is it concerned with service provision (e.g. is the department wasting money through inefficiencies?)?
- *Project objectives*: Do the objectives for the audit reflect both the reason the audit is being carried out and what the audit aims to achieve?
- *Whom to involve*: clinical staff, those implementing the change, managers, and so forth.
- *Standards for audit*: National Institute for Health and Care Excellence guidelines, research papers, professional organisation advice (royal colleges and so forth), a new standard created for this audit (e.g. the use of cheaper anti-emetics in acute care – there is not a 'standard' but this could cut costs dramatically).
- *Project plan*: What is to be audited? How big should the sample size be? Which cases should be investigated? What time period should be covered? Do you need further advice or involvement of statisticians or research fellows? Do you need ethics approval?
- *Action plan*: How are you to collect the data?
- *Pilot audit*: a trial run of the audit to highlight problems with data collection.

After the audit has been conducted and the results analysed, it is important to identify areas for improvement and to present these results to those who are able to implement the changes suggested. Areas to cover here include the following points.

- *Analysis of audit data*: make sure the results are accurate, complete and unbiased.
- *Presenting the results*: To whom? Those who will deliver the changes? Those in charge of the service?
- A *strategy for change*: How can shortcomings in practice be changed? Come up with ideas of how to create a better method for maintaining excellence in clinical care.
- *Implementing change*: Ensure those who are implementing the changes are aware of what they need to do. Make sure you have the backing of managers and senior staff. Continue to advertise the importance of the changes.

Finally, it is crucial to re-audit, otherwise you may simply have found a problem, come up with a change but not actually changed practice. If you re-audit, you are able to see if your proposed changes have been implemented and whether this has improved patient outcomes or service provision.

CHAPTER 13

R: research

TYPES OF RESEARCH

There are many different types of research, ranging from audits and case reports to randomised, controlled trials and systematic reviews. Some types of research are obviously easier to organise and participate in than others, but, if possible, it is still important to carry out a range of different types of research.

Some research is considered to be of a higher standard than others (the pyramid of research evidence), and while research from the top of the pyramid looks a lot better than from the bottom, it is much easier to get involved with and carry out types of research from the bottom of the pyramid. In this chapter you will find a very brief outline of the different types of research (for more information *see* Chapter 17, 'How to conduct research and publish your work').

Ideas, opinions and letters

It is relatively easy to get good letters and opinion pieces published in a journal. Even conversations had over dinner or in the pub can be developed into good letters and opinion pieces if written well. Try to target these to current issues and hot topics in medicine or the media to give them a higher impact. They do not have to be long and they can pose or try to answer ethical or controversial questions, drawing in replies from people who read the journal.

Case reports

Case reports have become increasingly difficult to get published because of the high volume of submissions journals receive in the form of case reports. However, this should not put you off. If you see an interesting, rare or difficult case, ask your consultant if it may be appropriate for writing up as a case report. To make a good case report there needs to be an important learning point that the case can be focused on. If you are finding it difficult to get a case report accepted, there is the option of paying to have it published in *BMJ Case Reports*. Ask your local hospital, medical school or NHS library first, as many will have subscriptions to this already, so that you do not have to pay to get your case report published.

Other types of research

There are many other types of research, as discussed in Chapter 17, which include case series, case-control studies and cohort studies. These are all different types of research whereby the publication is 'original research', but the detail of the methodologies is beyond the scope of this book.

Randomised, controlled trials and randomised, controlled, double-blind trials

These will be difficult to get involved with, as they will mostly be consultant led and will consist of multi-centre data collections. However, if you are offered the opportunity to become involved with one of these then, time permitting, you should always accept the opportunity, as it is an excellent thing to have on your CV.

Systematic reviews and meta-analyses

Systematic reviews and meta-analyses are the highest level of research. They are usually very time intensive and often require multiple authors to simply make the effort manageable. That said, they are more accessible for those 'lower down' the profession who are unable to conduct or become involved with randomised, controlled trials.

HOW TO START A RESEARCH PROJECT

If you are unsure how best to start and approach a research project, then talk with your registrar. Even if your registrar is not involved with research him- or herself, he or she may be able to point you in the direction of someone who is. Letters, opinion pieces and case reports can be written without your registrar's support, but it will be difficult to start up your own research project in the form of research further up the pyramid of evidence without his or her input and support.

First of all, come up with a question, preferably in an area that interests you. If it interests you then you are less likely to become disheartened with the work to be done. Discuss this question with a registrar or consultant and discuss how best to set up and collect the data needed.

Ethical approval

Ethics approval can be difficult to get and can take a long time. Speak to someone who has experience of applying for ethics approval, as this may mean you get approval first attempt rather than having to modify the application and try again. Make sure you apply as early as possible for ethics approval, as it can be a long and drawn-out process. Starting ethics applications early will mean that your research is not delayed, as you cannot start the data collection until you have ethics approval.

Conducting the research

Conducting the research is covered in much greater depth in Chapter 17, but the basics include making sure you adhere to the methodology, ensuring you abide by all ethical constraints, and at all times being scrupulously honest about your actions. There is nothing more useless than a research article that does not follow the methodology, as this can at best cloud the evidence base and at worst lead to adverse patient outcomes when someone bases a decision on your work.

Publication and presentation

Even after all that work there is still no guarantee that you will get the article accepted by a journal. However, if it is rejected by a journal, do not give up – try again and again to different journals. It is very likely that if the project is well designed and well thought out, it will eventually be accepted somewhere. If you are unable to find a journal that will accept it, try submitting it to a conference as a poster or presentation instead. This way you still get recognition for your work and it looks just as good on a CV. This is covered in greater depth in Chapter 18, 'How to present your research'.

SUMMARY

With any work you do, you should always try to get the most out of it – submit for publication as well as posters and presentations to ensure that your hard work does not go to waste. This will ensure that what you do improves both your learning and your career prospects and, eventually, it may improve patient care.

CHAPTER 14

K: knowledge

The knowledge aspect of the portfolio is concerned with the myriad ways of demonstrating what you know. The majority of things that you do in this respect are examinations. By graduating from medical school, you show that you have enough knowledge to practise safely and effectively as a Foundation trainee. However, as you progress through your career, it is not simply enough to have a medical degree. Examinations for the postgraduate colleges (such as the Royal College of Physicians) have membership exams, leading to qualifications such as the MRCP(UK). These examinations are known as 'gatekeeper' exams, as success in these is required to progress to the higher levels of training.

In this chapter, the main examinations are discussed and their general structure outlined. It is not possible to discuss every postgraduate examination, nor is it pertinent to discuss every fellowship examination. To this end, the membership examinations for anaesthetics, general practice, medicine, paediatrics, surgery, and obstetrics and gynaecology are discussed. However, the main structure is similar for most examinations, with written and practical examinations combined to produce the end result for the candidate. For more information on examinations not mentioned here, simply visit the relevant college's website and see their examinations page.

FELLOWSHIP OF THE ROYAL COLLEGE OF ANAESTHETISTS

The Fellowship of the Royal College of Anaesthetists (FRCA) examinations are made up of the Primary FRCA and the Final FRCA.

The Primary FRCA has two components: (1) an examination of multiple-choice questions (MCQs) and (2) both an OSCE and a structured oral examination (SOE). In order to be eligible to take the FRCA examination you must be a UK trainee in anaesthetics, the Acute Care Common Stem Programme or the Foundation Programme (MCQ section only) or be an anaesthetist. Once you have passed the Primary FRCA you have 7 years to take and pass the Final FRCA. You are only allowed five attempts at the MCQ paper and only four attempts at the OSCE and SOE.

The Final FRCA consists of a written paper and a SOE. The Final written paper is formed of MCQs and short-answer questions and you are only allowed six attempts at this examination. In order to be eligible to take this examination you must have passed the Primary FRCA within the last 7 years and you must be a trainee in anaesthetics.

The Final SOE consists of two sections: (1) clinical anaesthetics and (2) clinical science. In both of these sections clinical scenarios will be provided and set questions will be asked. Again, you only have six attempts in order to pass the Final SOE and you must have passed the Final written paper within the last 2 years in order to be able to take the Final SOE.

The Royal College of Anaesthetists advises that trainees discuss with their trainers and supervisors regarding when they will be best prepared for taking the examinations, so that limited attempts are not used up by taking the examinations at too early a stage in training.

MEMBERSHIP OF THE ROYAL COLLEGE OF GENERAL PRACTITIONERS

The Membership of the Royal College of General Practitioners (MRCGP) examinations have three parts: (1) the Applied Knowledge Test, (2) the Clinical Skills Assessment (CSA) and (3) workplace-based assessments.

You are eligible to take the Applied Knowledge Test once you are in ST2 or ST3 of the general practice training programme. You are limited to four attempts at this examination. This examination is designed to assess your knowledge base and it underpins general practice in the UK. It is a 3-hour computer-based test with 200 questions.

You are able to take the CSA once in the ST3 year of the general practice training programme and you are again limited to only four attempts at this examination. The CSA takes on the well-known OSCE format, with 13 10-minute stations. This examination is designed to test a wide variety of clinical and consultation skills.

The workplace-based assessments are designed to support your development and to highlight any areas of difficulty that need further work. There are a variety of different workplace-based assessments that are also used in other training programmes. Specific workplace-based assessment requirements can change from year to year and so it is wise to stay up to date with the information on the MRCGP website regarding these requirements.

It is recommended that candidates consider the timing of the examinations carefully with the educational and clinical supervisors to ensure that they do not apply to take the examinations too early thereby resulting in failed attempts.

MEMBERSHIP OF THE ROYAL COLLEGE OF OBSTETRICIANS AND GYNAECOLOGISTS

The Membership of the Royal College of Obstetricians and Gynaecologists (MRCOG) examination has two parts.

The Part 1 MRCOG consists of two written papers: Paper 1 covers the theory behind the specialty, including anatomy, genetics, endocrinology and epidemiology; Paper 2 covers clinical management, data interpretation, pathology and pharmacology, among other things. You are allowed unlimited attempts at the Part 1 examination and are encouraged to take it only after some experience in an obstetrics and gynaecology training post.

The Part 2 MRCOG consists of a written examination and an oral examination. The written examination must be passed prior to taking the oral examination. The oral examination consists of 12 stations that are a mixture of history taking, communication and clinical skills. Candidates may also be expected to critically appraise pieces of work in discussion with the examiner.

Candidates must have completed 2 years in an obstetrics and gynaecology training post following successful completion of Part 1 before they can be eligible to take Part 2. You have to at least have attempted Part 2 within 10 years of passing Part 1. You do not have to have passed Part 2 within this time frame, but if you do not attempt it you will be required to resit part 1.

MEMBERSHIP OF THE ROYAL COLLEGE OF PAEDIATRICS AND CHILD HEALTH

The Membership of the Royal College of Paediatrics and Child Health (MRCPCH) examinations changed format in 2013. This section will cover the new examination format.

The MRCPCH examinations have three parts: Part 1, Part 2 and the clinical. MRCPCH Part 1 involves two written examinations: part 1a, the MRCPCH Foundation of Practice paper, and part 1b, the MRCPCH Theory and Science paper. The MRCPCH Foundation of Practice paper focuses on the areas of child health important to those working with children in their medical careers. The MRCPCH Theory and Science paper focuses on the basic scientific, physiological and pharmacological principles upon which clinical practice is based. Both part 1a and part 1b consist of a mixture of extended matching questions and MCQs. The RCPCH recommends that you wait until you have had at least 6 months' experience in a paediatrics training post until you attempt MRCPCH Part 1; however, this is not a requirement. You can attempt MRCPCH Part 1 as many times as necessary in order to pass.

MRCPCH Part 2 is an examination of clinical knowledge and decision-making in all areas of paediatrics and child health. This again consists of two papers and will also include questions on research, audits, ethics and medical science applied to clinical care. There is no limit to attempts at the MRCPCH Part 2 examinations, and you have 7 years from passing MRCPCH Part 1 to pass and complete MRCPCH Part 2.

The clinical examination is aimed at assessing whether you have reached the standard of a newly appointed specialty registrar in clinical skills. The examination takes an OSCE format and has 10 stations. You must have passed both MRCPCH Part 1 and MRCPCH Part 2 in order to be eligible to take the clinical examination and you must have held your basic medical qualification for a minimum of 2½ years, with a minimum of 12 months spent in a post with exposure to dealing with paediatric emergencies. The Royal College of Paediatrics and Child Health has recently relaxed the ruling of three attempts only at the clinical examinations and candidates are now allowed as many attempts as needed within the 7-year period from passing the MRCPCH Part 1 examinations.

MEMBERSHIP OF THE ROYAL COLLEGES OF PHYSICIANS OF THE UNITED KINGDOM

The MRCP(UK) examinations consist of Part 1, Part 2 written and PACES (the clinical examination).

You are not permitted to apply to take the MRCP(UK) examinations until you have been graduated for a minimum of 12 months and have successfully completed at least 1 year of training in a medical post (i.e. FY1). There is no restriction to the number of times that you can sit MRCP(UK) Part 1 in order to pass. Once you have successfully passed you will have 7 years from the date of the examination to complete all other parts of the MRCP examinations.

MRCP(UK) Part 1 is aimed at testing your broad knowledge base and your ability to apply this knowledge to common and important medical disorders as well as clinical science.

MRCP(UK) Part 2 written is aimed at showing that you have the minimum level of knowledge required for a physician in training and that you are able to apply this knowledge to clinical situations, using clinical reasoning and problem-solving.

PACES are the clinical exams designed to test your clinical knowledge and skills, aimed at ensuring that you can provide a high level of care to your patients.

Candidates who have successfully completed MRCP(UK) Part 1 are eligible to apply to take MRCP(UK) Part 2 written and MRCP(UK) Part 2 clinical (also known as 'PACES') examinations. You are allowed six attempts at the MRCP(UK) Part 2 written and MRCP(UK) Part 2 clinical (PACES) examinations but your educational supervisor must support each application.

The Royal Colleges of Physicians recommends that you are unlikely to be successful in your attempt to pass the MRCP(UK) Part 2 examinations until you have completed your 2-year Foundation Programme and have started the Core Training Programme (*see* Figure 14.1). However, you are unable to progress to ST3 training programmes and above without having completed the MRCP(UK), so you need to plan ahead to ensure that you are able to complete all examinations prior to interviews and the end of the core training years.

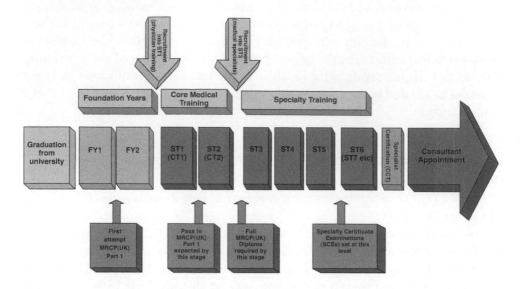

FIGURE 14.1 The 'standard' career pathway in medical careers, with examples of when to sit each aspect of the MRCP(UK) examination, Specialty Certificate Examination (SCE) and Certificate of Completion of Training (CCT).

MEMBERSHIP OF THE ROYAL COLLEGE OF SURGEONS

The Membership of the Royal College of Surgeons examination (MRCS) consists of MRCS Part A and MRCS Part B.

MRCS Part A is a written MCQ examination made up of two 2-hour papers: (1) Applied Basic Sciences and (2) Principles of Surgery-in-General. Both papers are sat on the same day and you must pass each individual paper as well as achieve the overall pass mark. You are allowed as many attempts at MRCS Part A as you need in order to pass.

MRCS Part B is an OSCE and usually consists of 18 stations, each lasting 9 minutes. These stations are made up of a combination of anatomy and surgical pathology, applied surgical science and critical care, communication skills in giving and receiving information and history taking, as well as clinical and procedural skills. A number of the stations will be examined in the context of your chosen specialty and this choice must be indicated upon application for the examination. It is important to know that only four attempts are allowed to pass MRCS Part B and so it is important not to disadvantage yourself by applying to take the examinations too early before you have adequate experience.

The Royal College of Surgeons advises that MRCS Part A is taken in ST1/CT1 and MRCS Part B is taken in ST2/CT2. However, many people start the examinations in their Foundation years by taking MRCS Part A and then wait until they have had further experience in order to take MRCS Part B.

SUMMARY

There are examinations for every specialty, and details of these examinations can easily be found on the relevant website. It is important to be aware of what the examinations consist of prior to applying for them and to also be aware of any time or attempt limits applying to the different exams. While many people will rush into taking the examinations in order to look good on their CV, it can put you at a disadvantage if you use one of your limited attempts at an examination by taking the examination too early and failing. It is always useful to have a good period of experience in the chosen specialty prior to attempting the examinations, as you are then more likely to pass successfully on your first attempt. Another thought should be towards cost and benefit – these examinations are not free and most cost upwards of £400. Therefore, sitting these too early may be a waste of money as well as a waste of your time and a waste of a valuable examination attempt.

FURTHER READING

- The Royal College of Anaesthetists: www.rcoa.ac.uk/examinations
- The Royal College of General Practitioners: www.rcgp.org.uk/gp-training-and-exams/mrcgp-exam-overview.aspx
- The Royal College of Obstetricians and Gynaecologists: www.rcog.org.uk/education-and-exams/examinations
- Royal College of Paediatrics and Child Health: www.rcpch.ac.uk/training-examinations-professional-development/assessment-and-examinations/assessment-and-examination
- Membership of the Royal Colleges of Physicians of the United Kingdom: www.mrcpuk.org/Pages/Home.aspx
- The Royal College of Surgeons of England: www.rcseng.ac.uk/exams

CHAPTER 15

E: education

EDUCATION OPPORTUNITIES

An expected part of being a doctor is that you will teach both your colleagues and your juniors, who will be the future of the profession. Without colleagues teaching colleagues, none of us would be able to continue the lifelong learning that is so crucial to being a part of the medical profession.

MEDICAL STUDENTS TEACHING MEDICAL STUDENTS

There are multiple opportunities at medical school to teach fellow medical students, whether it is formal, supported teaching or opportunistic teaching to help a fellow student with examination revision.

Many medical schools still teach anatomy in the dissection room, recruiting medical students from older years to teach the younger years. This would be a structured, supported teaching opportunity where you would be able to provide supervised teaching as well as receive feedback not only from the students you are teaching but also from staff members. This opportunity would also allow you to consolidate your own learning of anatomy, ensuring that you revisit knowledge learnt earlier in the course.

It may not always be possible to become involved with structured teaching opportunities such as those described. The demand will be high, with a lot of people wanting to participate in order to improve their CVs. However, opportunistic teaching to fellow medical students either on the ward, or as revision help for exams, will allow you to hone and improve your teaching techniques and receive feedback as to how to improve your teaching style. While this will not count as teaching experience for interviews or CVs, it will benefit you in the long run, as you will have practice at teaching.

FOUNDATION DOCTORS TEACHING MEDICAL STUDENTS

The majority of hospitals these days play host to medical students from various universities, which provides valuable teaching opportunities for Foundation doctors. If you are aware of medical students in the hospital in which you are working, then contact the local medical school coordinators and volunteer to get involved with teaching. This is also the perfect chance to offer to set up a teaching programme if one does not already exist.

Setting up a teaching programme for medical students can easily be done. Most junior doctors are eager to be involved with teaching, so volunteers to run sessions should not be a problem. Liaising with the medical students themselves in order to ensure that teaching sessions are at a convenient time and are on relevant and helpful topics for them is important in order to make sure that your teaching programme is a success.

If there is already a teaching programme in place, ensure that the person organising it has your contact details and knows that you are keen to be involved. Always prepare teaching sessions well in advance to ensure that they are structured, organised and interesting for the students.

It is also important to make time for medical students on the ward. While your jobs will be busy and hectic, think back to your time at medical school and you will probably remember that the best teaching sessions happened opportunistically on the wards with junior doctors. As Foundation doctors you are in a perfect position to remember what it was like studying for medical school exams, and what knowledge and skills are important and necessary to know at medical school. As you progress through your medical career you will become more detached from what it was like to be a medical student and what knowledge was necessary and what was not. Opportunistic teaching on the ward is important for practising and honing practical skills and techniques; it is important not only for medical students but also for junior doctors to receive such teaching from their seniors.

REGISTRARS STARTING JOURNAL CLUBS AND TEACHING SESSIONS

It is important for teaching to continue throughout your medical career. As you progress up the career ladder it is important that the type of teaching that you participate in changes and evolves. While it is still important to participate in opportunistic teaching of both medical students and more junior doctors on the wards, it is also important to organise more structured teaching sessions, such as journal clubs.

FORMAL AND INFORMAL TEACHING

Bedside teaching or ward round tuition to medical students is an ideal time to share your knowledge and practise your teaching skills; however, almost all people applying for jobs are well versed in this form of teaching. In fact, the majority of good candidates will begin their answer to a teaching-related interview question with something along the lines of: '*As well as the numerous informal teaching sessions and opportunities that I have undertaken as a part of my day-to-day work, I have also ...*'. This shows that they are always thinking about teaching in their daily routine and that they are aware of how important this is to everyday medicine and improving the quality of the next crop of doctors.

The majority of hospitals hosting Foundation trainees will also have medical students. This gives you the opportunity to undertake teaching and develop your teaching skills on a relatively tame and enthusiastic audience. If this is the case, ensure you take part in the teaching programme for students, and if there is no programme running at present, offer to organise this.

Teaching scores a great number of points on applications, but only for formal teaching. The points scored are lowest for those who just partake in the odd teaching session, they increase for those organising local courses and they are highest for those who are members of the faculty on a teaching course.

TEACHING COURSES

There are often teaching courses organised by each deanery. These are specifically aimed at doctors in training posts who want to begin to learn about how to effectively teach across a wide range of situations.

Many universities and teaching hospitals run 'training the trainers' courses. Many of the royal colleges also run these courses, with the aim of deepening the understanding of how people learn so that educators can plan, deliver, evaluate and develop training and teaching in a more effective way. Attending one of these courses can be expensive; however, attending and gaining a certificate of having completed the course means that you will be more likely to be selected to deliver teaching to both students and junior doctors if there is competition for the teaching posts.

FEEDBACK AND CERTIFICATES

Feedback is crucial for teaching: without it, teachers do not get better, the courses do not evolve, and those lessons that are excellent may not get repeated, while those that are not well taught are not highlighted as needing improvement.

The need for feedback is the first on the list: the teachers do not get better. Here, you can use feedback as a means of guiding your reflective practice. You may present five lectures, with four getting full marks and the fifth getting poor feedback. With the feedback you will know that this lecture needs improving and you may want to approach medical education experts for help. Without the feedback it can be easy to assume you have got better with the experience of teaching.

Feedback also provides a form of evidence that the teaching session actually took place. This is important, as it demonstrates that several people have attended your lecture and have taken the time to give the feedback. This is a vital part of your portfolio, enabling your portfolio assessors to see how others perceive your teaching style, what you are good at, and what you are not as good at. For example, some people are excellent at teaching theoretical knowledge but not at teaching practical skills. Here feedback brings this to light and either allows the teacher to specialise in theoretical teaching, or to attend courses and improve his or her practical skills teaching. This, again, is another form of 'demonstrating reflection and self-improvement', which, if you can get your assessor or interviewer to think that this is something that you are continually doing in your day-to-day practice, you will score the maximal points in any application for this station.

CHAPTER 16

T: training

There is very little more core to medicine than training. This is started on your first day of medical school and continues until the day you retire. Without training, you have no means of improving your skills other than reading and experience. While these are excellent means of consolidating knowledge and are potentially capable of producing small volumes of skills and knowledge, training is crucial to developing as a doctor.

Maintaining clinical skills is something that every doctor is required to do by the GMC to retain his or her licence to practise medicine. However, it is very difficult to prove that you do this without undergoing training. Every doctor will read and every doctor will gain experience, but to maintain an excellent standard of practice, as every doctor should aspire to, training is required.

With training, experts in areas come together to treat novices, trainees or experts from other areas in their particular skill set. This ranges from registrars and consultants teaching clinical skills at their local medical school, to cardiothoracic surgeons discussing the latest in standalone thoracoscopic atrial fibrillation surgery with GPs and when this is appropriate. The range of what can be taught is vast, and it is simply not possible to discuss every training course here, but the main types of training course are discussed in this chapter. Gaining experience of training courses early in your career is good practice, as it shows that you are both keen to improve and able to learn in this environment, as well as enabling you to become familiar and comfortable in these situations.

ROUTINE CLINICAL SKILLS TEACHING

Throughout your training, you will be taught to perform procedures. The old teaching adage of 'see one, do one, teach one' is essentially what this is describing. Here you will take a new skill, such as an ascitic drain, and watch a gastroenterology registrar perform this as he or she talks you through it. Then you will be asked to perform the same skill under the registrar's guidance and supervision. Following this, the registrar will observe you, but will not intervene unless necessary. Finally, you will then be asked to teach someone else, while the registrar observes and corrects any mistakes you make. It is felt that, following this process, you will be 'competent' to perform this procedure on your own. This can occur for many clinical skills, from a lumbar puncture to a 'femoral stab'. The outcome of this training is the completion of a DOPS (*see* Chapter 5, 'Core and run-through trainees') by the supervising doctor, which acts as proof that you have been trained in this procedure.

CLINICAL SKILLS TRAINING COURSES

Clinical skills training courses are completely different to routine clinical skills teaching, as you are not based in your usual environment. These are usually a combination of lectures and practical sessions, where the lectures give you the theoretical knowledge to carry out the skill both effectively and safely, while alerting you to the potential side effects (e.g. bowel perforation in an ascitic drain).

The practical sessions allow you to perform this skill for the first time in a safe, calm and enabling atmosphere on models or animal cadavers. This allows you room for error and means that you are able to discuss what you are doing, asking questions as you go, which may not be appropriate for clinical scenarios – imagine your doctors asking, '*So which needle do I use to put into the patient's spine?*'!

The culmination of clinical skills training courses is an assessment and, if you pass this, a certificate of competence. This then shows that you are able to perform this procedure when you return to work.

CLINICAL APPROACH TRAINING COURSES

'Clinical approach' is a term that encompasses many different training courses. Here you are taught how to approach a particular scenario or group of scenarios in clinical practice. An example is the Care of the Critically Ill Surgical Patient course of the Royal College of Surgeons. This course aims to teach surgeons a safe and systematic way of approaching their unwell patients to ensure the best outcomes for the patients. The course will run through multiple scenarios and by the end will not only have endowed the participants with the knowledge required to deal with the most common problems affecting surgical patients but also have bestowed a sensible method for approaching those patients who do not fall into the scenarios taught.

Again, at the end of the course, participants who pass the assessment are awarded a certificate of clinical competence. This does not say you are able to perform a particular procedure, but that you are competent to work in these situations and that you are more able to deal with problems when they arise in clinical practice.

Some of these courses are mandatory for progression to the next stage of your career, such as advanced life support, advanced trauma life support, and so forth.

SPECIALTY-SPECIFIC TRAINING PROGRAMMES

There are far too many specialty-specific training programmes available for doctors to attend them all, but you should be aware of their existence, as they may be a requirement for you to move to the next stage of your career, or they can act as a great means of showing commitment to your specialty. The royal colleges usually deal with these training programmes and you should visit their websites for more information.

Section 4

How to publish your work

'Publish or perish' – the words often muttered by consultants and those giving advice on how to ensure you progress with your career. While this may sound like a nice rhyme with little substance, there is a definite underlying message at its core. Yes, it is most certainly possible to make it through a round of competition without publishing, especially for Foundation year applications. However, as you progress through the hierarchy of medical grades to core training and specialty training, it soon becomes apparent that publications are increasingly important and that there will be many people around you that are published, and you have to catch up these marks on your application elsewhere.

Publishing can have varying levels of usefulness for an application. When you are a medical student, any form of publication is an excellent achievement. As you progress through to Foundation training, you should aim to become more 'generally specific'; that is, once you have decided upon, for example, surgery, then you should aim to publish within one of the surgical disciplines to improve your chances of gaining a core surgical training post. Once you have your core training post, you should aim to publish in a highly specific manner – you should aim to write articles that are based around the specific specialty into which you are hoping to progress.

Publishing can take many forms, from full journal articles that most are familiar with, through case reports and correspondence articles, to posters and presentations at conferences. This section will provide useful information to allow you to understand the basics of the different types of publication as well as constructive tips on how to improve your chances of getting published.

CHAPTER 17

How to conduct research and publish your work

Dr Joseph M Norris

ACADEMIC FOUNDATION YEAR 1 DOCTOR

Why bother writing a paper? Why not take up extreme frisbee, follow beach volleyball or go to a party? The truth is, writing and publishing is integral to all of medicine and science. Not only is it the primary medium for conveying your work to others, so that they may learn, utilise and build upon it, but it is also something you must do if you are to make the most of your medical career. As the old adage goes *'Publish or perish'*.

Despite this, writing is something that few medical students and junior doctors know how to do, especially without neglecting their studies or patients. Surprisingly, publishing is a domain that medical schools utterly neglect from their curricula and medical schools and deaneries must address this in the near future.

Increasing emphasis is placed upon producing papers and this can cause enormous stress to students. Pressure increases at each competitive career juncture, so it is imperative to get to grips with publishing now. In the UK, several 'points' are awarded to students for publications when applying to the Foundation Programme for their first jobs as junior doctors. Further credit is given to students applying to the Academic Foundation Programme, for multiple papers, varying article types and author positions.

Obviously, before getting published, you are going to have to write a paper! But how to do this? Probably the most important facet to consider is what type of paper to publish. This chapter will sequentially consider each article type, with appropriate writing tips. It won't teach how to 'do science' – this is learnt elsewhere. Rather, this chapter is intended to give an introduction on how to put science down on paper.

The main categories of paper in biomedicine are original articles, review articles, case reports, correspondence articles and miscellaneous articles. Before discussing each category, it is pertinent to consider unifying features: titles, abstracts and key words.

TITLES, ABSTRACTS AND KEY WORDS
Titles

An effective title can make or break a paper. As with most things in life, titles must be balanced. On the one hand, a title must succinctly summarise the paper, without overstating the content. On the other hand, a title must be well phrased and stylish, so as to grab the reader's attention and draw him or her in. Remember, obey given journal formatting and be as descriptive and specific as possible – for instance, state whether the study was prospective, randomised, laboratory based or multi-centred. Read a dozen paper titles in your journal of choice and you'll get a grasp of their overall form. One final piece of advice: avoid acronyms and abbreviations – these really upset reviewers.

Abstracts

An abstract is a précis of your work. Abstracts are found in most articles, except correspondence, as the correspondence format is too terse to warrant them. For everything else, including submissions for conference posters and presentations, you are going to have to write an abstract. They are arguably the most important part of a paper, especially following the advent of electronic journals and search engines. Put simply, abstracts contain core, distilled information in as succinct a paragraph as possible. They are usually 200–300 words long and take one of two forms: structured or unstructured.

Br J Ophthalmol. 2005 Aug;89(8):956-9.

Imaging of osteo-odonto-keratoprosthesis by electron beam tomography.

Fong KC[1], Ferrett CG, Tandon R, Paul B, Herold J, Liu CS.

Abstract
AIM: To describe the experience of using electron beam tomography (EBT) in imaging of osteo-odonto-keratoprosthesis (OOKP) to identify early bone and dentine loss which may threaten the viability of the eye.

METHODS: Seven patients with an OOKP in one eye underwent EBT. The OOKP lamina dimensions were measured on EBT and compared to the manual measurements at the time of surgery.

RESULTS: There was a high degree of resolution of the OOKP lamina noted with EBT. In particular, it identified three patients with a marked degree of thinning of the lamina edges. Two of these patients had OOKP that were allografts. The mean time from surgery to examination was 3.6 years (range 1.2-5 years) while the mean age of the patients was 56 years (range 31-79 years).

CONCLUSIONS: It is important to monitor regularly the dimensions and stability of the OOKP lamina as it will help detect cases that are at risk of extrusion of the optical cylinder and consequent endophthalmitis. Prophylactic measures can then be taken to prevent such serious complications from occurring. In this series, the authors found EBT to have excellent resolution and speed and they would support regular scanning of the OOKP lamina in all patients.

FIGURE 17.1 An example of a structured abstract from the *British Journal of Ophthalmology*[1]

Structured abstracts (*see* Figure 17.1) are easy to write, so as long as you follow author guidelines meticulously (a golden rule in publishing). Journals tend to have a set of strict rules for authors; these should be the first thing that you track down before writing your paper – there is no point carefully writing an article that is unsuitable for publication! The 'structure' usually consists of aim, methods, results and conclusions (or similar variant); only write a sentence or two for each of these sections. Make sure sentences are 'content rich' – that is, that they contain most salient background features and your most statistically significant results.

Unstructured abstracts (*see* Figure 17.2) can be harder to write, as *you* have to decide what to include. A piece of advice: follow what other authors have done for your intended journal; such abstracts are easy to locate, as PubMed is littered with them. As a general rule, an unstructured abstract will follow the same format as a structured one, without specified headings. One slight variation of content is that unstructured abstracts do not normally open with a blunt declaration of study aims. Other than that, all previous advice is applicable.

J Vasc Surg. 2012 Aug;56(2):486-8. doi: 10.1016/j.jvs.2012.01.064. Epub 2012 Mar 9.

Bilateral popliteal artery aneurysms in a young man with Loeys-Dietz syndrome.

Stephenson MA[1], Vlachakis I, Valenti D.

Abstract

Loeys-Dietz syndrome is a recently described genetic connective tissue disorder. The syndrome is associated with multiple nonvascular phenotypic anomalies but also aggressive arteriopathy, which has so far principally been shown to cause aortic root dilatation with subsequent dissection and rupture. We report the first ever case of a young man diagnosed with Loeys-Dietz syndrome with asymptomatic large bilateral popliteal artery aneurysms. We have successfully resected these aneurysms and revascularized with synthetic graft.

FIGURE 17.2 An example of an unstructured abstract from the *Journal of Vascular Surgery*[2]

Key words

The majority of articles have a rarely discussed feature: *key words*. These are written directly after the abstract, and so here seems an appropriate place to discuss them. Key words are usually five to ten words that most pertinently summarise your article. It is up to you which key words you choose and, while they're not crucial for success, it is worth choosing words that are appropriate and searchable.

The following are three key points about key words.

1. They should be searchable within the Medical Subject Headings (or MeSH) database (available at: www.nlm.nih.gov/mesh). Obviously this isn't always feasible, particularly if you're describing something novel for the first time, but wherever possible you should do this, as it will result in correct search-linking in PubMed.
2. Words should be written in alphabetical order. Some journals specify this and others don't. It is safest to stick with this simple rule though.
3. Separate key words with a semicolon. Capital letter for the first. No punctuation after the last. Easy.

> **TOP TIP**
>
> Make your abstract attractive. Use snappy sentences with the occasional jazzy word to dazzle the editor (be very tactful about this). Include your most important findings and state with total lucidity how these are adding to the literature.

ORIGINAL ARTICLES

These papers are the real deal. Original articles are the staple currency of scientific writing and are given highest precedence. All major pieces of research are presented in original articles and take an accepted format. To write an original article, you will need to have undertaken a scientific study; for this reason, original articles are probably the hardest for medical students and junior doctors to publish. They are also worth the most for job applications and in the view of your seniors. Writing an original article can be challenging, so it is worth knowing their general format. Broadly, they follow the structure outlined in the following list.

1. *Introduction*. Keep this simple. The introduction should begin confidently with a short sentence or two outlining the relevant background to the study. Then, another sentence should be given describing the hypothesis, followed by a final sentence summarising experimental methodology. Don't overdo this, and remember to only use around three to four references, across the three or four sentences.

2. *Methods*. In theory, an experimenter should be able to 'recreate' a study by reading this section. In reality, the methods should not be an overly detailed scientific 'recipe' but, rather, a statement of patient demographics, cohort size and any study-specific methodology. Reviewers also like to see study duration, control selection, inclusion criteria, exclusion criteria, outcome measures, whether tools or questionnaires have been validated, *who* undertook the investigation and the respective degree of blinding. When alluding to previously described tools, you should provide a reference. Usually, a comment on statistics is given, ideally describing *what* statistics package was used to interrogate the data, *which* tests were used and *how* power was calculated (if it was).

3. *Results*. Results should be listed logically, with complementary tables and figures, allowing readers to grasp the main points without having to do excessive reading. Nevertheless, avoid undue repetition between tables and text. Information in the results section should correlate with that given in the methods, in terms of patients, outcomes and tests.

4. *Discussion*. The discussion allows you to really open the paper up and draw in more references. Resist the temptation to go over the top and maintain focus to the original central hypothesis, without introducing bias when interpreting results. Separate paragraphs can be dedicated to each identifiable issue or implication, with appropriate reference to relevant studies. Strictly speaking, limitations should be detailed at the end of the discussion

section but it would be wise not to overdo this – you don't want to shoot your paper down!

5. *Conclusion*. Finish the paper in style, summarising standout findings, implications for future research, how relevant and original the study is, whether it is concordant with previous findings and whether there are controversial ramifications.

6. *Acknowledgements*. Not a deal-clincher, but it is polite and proper to thank all those who have helped with the study but have not contributed sufficiently for authorship.

7. *References*. References must be listed meticulously, in the given style of the journal (usually Vancouver referencing style). Reviewers do not usually have the time to assess accuracy, but it is wise to check this carefully before submission – it would be embarrassing to be rejected for inadequate or inaccurate referencing. There may even be the suggestion of one of the highest academic crimes – plagiarism – if referencing is not perfect.

TOP TIP

At the end of the day, the reviewers and editorial board decide whether or not to accept your paper. Your aim is to please them! Do this by stating how your results have advanced existing knowledge or practices. Follow their guidelines and be as concise as possible in each of the aforementioned sections.

REVIEW ARTICLES

Reviews are useful articles, summarising a particular subsection of the literature. They can take many forms, such as extensive and thorough systematic reviews, through to statistically rigorous meta-analyses. They are often long, with timely conclusions. Previously, reviews presented an opportunity for juniors to write a summary in conjunction with a senior and gain themselves a highly respected

Int J Oral Maxillofac Surg. 2012 Aug;41(8):885-94. doi: 10.1016/j.ijom.2012.04.024. Epub 2012 Jun 6.

Facial feminization surgery: current state of the art.

Altman K.

Abstract

Facial feminization surgery (FFS) is a group of surgical procedures; the objectives of which are to change the features of a male face to that of a female face. This surgery does not aim to rejuvenate the face. FFS is carried out almost exclusively on transsexual women (males who are transitioning into females) and who have gender dysphoria. Some non-transsexual women may undergo some feminizing surgical procedures if they feel that they have male facial characteristics. Most transsexual women will have lived in role for sometime and they often undergo FFS before any other form of gender reassignment surgery as it assists them in passing as a female and integrating into everyday society. Various specific facial surgical procedures are utilized to feminize the face, often involving sculpture and contouring of the facial skeleton. These include correction of the hairline by scalp advance, contouring the forehead, brow lift, rhinoplasty, cheek implants, resection of the buccal fat pads of Bichat, lip lift and lip augmentation with dermis graft, mandible angle reduction and taper, genioplasty and thyroid shave. This article discusses the current state of the art in facial feminization surgery.

FIGURE 17.3 An example of an expert review article from the *International Journal of Oral and Maxillofacial Surgery*[3]

paper. Unfortunately, in recent times, reviews have become seen as something that should only be written by an expert (*see* Figure 17.3). Indeed, such experts are regularly invited ('commissioned') to write reviews for journals on particular topics; commissions can be for standard or themed editions.

Ostensibly, review articles do not make a fantastic place for students and juniors to begin their foray into the publishing world. However, there are rare exceptions. There is a new format of review that debutant authors can write successfully: Best Evidence Topic (BestBET) reviews. These take a very particular format, answering a narrow clinical question. Relevant databases are carefully searched for existing evidence and papers that rank most highly on the Oxford Centre for Evidence-Based Medicine Levels of Evidence are selected. From these papers, outcome measures and results relevant to the original clinical question are extracted, tabulated and compared to form a consensus clinical bottom line. BestBET articles are beginning to spread in medicine and it would be worth reading the *Emergency Medical Journal, Interactive Cardiovascular and Thoracic Surgery* or the *International Journal of Surgery* for an introduction to the genre.

TOP TIP

When writing a BestBET, run the clinical question by a registrar or a consultant in that specialty. There is no point breaking a sweat over a topic that is not even worth the 'paper' it is written on.

CASE REPORTS

A case report is a short summary of an interesting or rare case delivered concisely, with a review of the pertinent literature. Previously, case reports were *the* first port of call for all budding academic medics. In recent years this has come under question, with increasing numbers of journals either refusing case reports altogether or having awfully low acceptance rates. Concurrently, and perhaps in response to this move, there has been an increase in the number of dedicated case-report-only journals. These focused journals present an apposite place to submit case reports, although they frequently have the drawback of charging steep publishing fees for open access.

You will need to find a case before writing it up. When delivering case presentations on the ward or at grand rounds, a senior might approach you and suggest that the case be written up; in these situations, it should be obvious when you have the germ of a good report. At other times, you'll have to be more on the ball to find your case. A good rule of thumb: if your consultant has not seen a condition before, then this is probably suitable for a case report! However, clinical interest and educational value take precedence over novelty or rarity in today's academic climate.

When writing the case up, stick to writing to inform rather than impress. Case reports take a relatively open format that allows you to discuss the diagnostic approach, context, clinical reasoning and patient outcome more freely. Be selective in details included from the clinical history and be sure that your discussion and literature review help justify your conclusions. Ideally, your literature review should reveal the paucity of information in your chosen niche – so that your place in the medical literature can be cemented.

Sadly, it can be difficult to get a case through to publication, thanks to the sheer volume submitted to journals. Here is a beautiful and evocative (if a little deflating) quote regarding case reports and their chance of being accepted by a journal for publication:

> But they are like birds tossed over a stormy ocean: only a few gain a foothold in the rigging of passing ships—for the rest, oblivion.[4]

TOP TIP

High-quality photography (or radiological or histopathological imaging) is essential. *A picture is worth a thousand words* – this is entirely true for case reports, and good images can secure an acceptance. Some specialties (such as dermatology) keep detailed clinical photography in patients' notes, making it easy to obtain photography. In other situations, it might be wise to carry a cheap digital camera in your bag, so that you never miss that crucial intra-operative shot.

CORRESPONDENCE

An apropos place to start for first-time writers is with correspondence articles or 'Letters to the Editor.' In summary, these articles are usually concise opinion pieces, in response to published research or as stand-alone pieces, discussing topical issues, or occasionally presenting research not substantial enough to warrant a full original article. They may not garner as much respect as a big review article or an original research paper, but they are easier for juniors to write and are often listed on major databases. It is pertinent to remember, though, that letters are considered opinion pieces and thus are the lowest form of evidence on the Oxford Centre for Evidence-Based Medicine Levels of Evidence ; as such, you must persistently aim to publish more substantial pieces.

Where to start: SPARK.

It may be tricky for the inexperienced to generate appropriate material for correspondence and so you may find the following mnemonic helpful. It might even light a SPARK of an idea for a letter.

S – Stay alert for grey areas, changing practice, future concepts and controversial opinions.

P – Published papers are easily mined, critiqued or added to. Authors deeply value feedback.

A – Attempt submission. There is nothing to lose. Responses are often quick and constructive.

R – Revise a rejected letter. They tend to be so short that tweaking is painless.

K – Keep going! Letters are important. If your idea is original and stimulating, it should get published.

TOP TIP

Take a 'dual pronged' approach to letter success. First, make some rough notes on a topic that you consider interesting or cutting-edge (but which you have no actual results or evidence for). Then search PubMed for a published article that is linked to your original thoughts. You can then publish your own thoughts in a *Letter to the Editor* of this journal – so long as you make some comment on the article that you have found!

MISCELLANEOUS ARTICLES

Several journal-specific articles exist, including editorials, technical tips and innumerable others. These offer potential avenues for juniors who have material that is unsuitable for other article types. The most difficult part of this type of article is not writing the article but, rather, actually knowing which subtypes exist.

Editorials are an unsuitable place for medical students and junior doctors to make their formative mark on the publishing world, as they are reserved for those in positions of seniority in journals, such as the editors. Such authors usually write monthly and are often professors and leaders of their field. So, while editorials are interesting to read, they are not appropriate to emulate during the early years.

Ann R Coll Surg Engl. 2005 May;87(3):211-2.

Orthopaedic instrument ideal for manual evacuation of faeces.

Moore EM.

FIGURE 17.4 An example of a technical tip article (without an abstract) from the *Annals of the Royal College of Surgeons of England* [5]

Technical tip articles are short, informative pieces that, in parallel with correspondence articles, do not usually have abstracts (*see* Figure 17.4). When you are on the ward or in theatre with a consultant and you hear him or her say,

'This is a little trick of my own that makes this particular pesky task a darn sight easier!' you should listen closely. Ask the consultant whether he or she has written the technique up, and then politely move in for the kill and see whether the consultant would mind if you wrote it up for him or her (with the consultant as senior author, obviously!). This is an easy way to gain technical tip articles – the key is to remain highly opportunistic.

Writing miscellaneous articles is similar to writing any other article; the same stylistic, grammatical and scientific laws still apply. It is vital to follow author guidelines, as these articles are really unique to each journal. They are normally shorter than original articles, but in rare cases they can be much longer. When writing niche articles, remember that they occasionally allow incorporation of audio and video, which can add real spice to your portfolio.

TOP TIP

Keep your eyes peeled for anything original. If a consultant says that he has invented a particular suturing technique, always ask whether you can write it up and submit it somewhere for him!

FINAL THOUGHTS

The following is a list of auxiliary topics and jargon that should be addressed.

- **Cover letter**. *Short letter to the Editor-in-Chief.* This letter should be brief but polite; emphasising why the editor should accept your work, that all authors are happy to submit the manuscript in its current form, and that it has not been simultaneously submitted elsewhere.
- **Authorship**. *Who has written the paper?* Generally speaking, the 'senior' author should go last and the author who has contributed most should go first. Make sure that everyone is clear as to his or her position before writing has begun, as this can be a tremendously thorny issue. One idea is to draft author names at the top of the paper from the outset of writing – so that everyone is 'on the same page'.
- **Journal choice**. *Choosing which journal to submit to can be difficult.* You must weigh up a number of factors. Obviously the high-impact factor journals are better for your CV and your career. On the flip side, you are less likely to have a paper accepted if you submit to the finest journals in the land, such as the *Lancet* or the *BMJ*.
- **Listing and databasing**. *Where your paper will be listed.* The most important database is PubMed. This is often *the* number-one thing that medical students worry about when considering submitting a paper to a journal. In the early stages of your career it is crucial to aim for journals that are listed on PubMed, as these are often the only ones that are acknowledged (e.g. for the Foundation Programme application).
- **Open-access**. *Free article access for readers.* A mixed blessing, this can cost a

lot to you as the author to publish (up to £2400, but usually in the range of £300 to £400), but it will massively increase visibility and thus citation rates, as more people are able to read your article for free.

- **Peer review**. *The acid test that articles must pass before publication*. This is the process by which 'peers' (other doctors and scientists) review your article, either blindly or non-blindly, to see whether it is of a high enough standard for publication. Once they have read the article, reviewers then make a decision: accept, reject, or accept with revision. The peer-review process is flawed, but it is the current gold standard method used all over the world.

SUMMARY

Publishing is amazingly satisfying and rewarding. When you have something to say in science, you should say it. Moreover, and nobody should be ashamed to admit this, *you need to publish to succeed*. It is to be hoped that this chapter has conveyed enthusiasm for this subject and outlined the issues surrounding the most important facet of publishing: writing the paper.

When writing your abstract, read guidelines carefully! Stick to the word count, make it structured or unstructured as required, select striking findings and use lively, to-the-point prose. For key words, follow three simple steps: (1) choose terms from the MeSH database, (2) set in alphabetical order and (3) use semicolons. It should now be clear which of the numerous article types is most suitable for your work. Original and review articles are tricky to publish at a junior stage; remember the possibilities that BestBETs hold though. Case reports and correspondence articles offer golden opportunities for students; all you need is a SPARK of an idea. Editorials are non-starters until you reach positions of seniority, but the assortment of miscellaneous articles represents multiple openings for publication – you just need to keep your eyes open, and then get searching for a suitable niche article type.

It is to be hoped that you will embrace the tips given in this chapter and go on to make a significant contribution to the scientific literature, thus immortalising your beautiful name. Writing and publishing is really not as hard as you think it is. So, what are you waiting for?

REFERENCES

1. Fong KC, Ferrett CG, Tandon R, *et al*. Imaging of osteo-odonto-keratoprosthesis by electron beam tomography. *Br J Ophthalmol*. 2005 Aug; **89**(8): 956–9.
2. Stephenson MA, Vlachakis I, Valenti D. Bilateral popliteal artery aneurysms in a young man with Loeys-Dietz syndrome. *J Vasc Surg*. 2012 Aug; **56**(2): 486–8.
3. Altman K. Facial feminization surgery: current state of the art. *Int J Oral Maxillofac Surg*. 2012 Aug; **41**(8): 885–94.
4. Fox R. Writing a case report: an editor's eye view. *Hosp Med*. 2000 Dec; **61**(12): 863–4.
5. Moore EM. Orthopaedic instrument ideal for manual evacuation of faeces. *Ann R Coll Surg Engl*. 2005 May; **87**(3): 211–12.

CHAPTER 18

How to present your research

Dr Meher Lad

FOUNDATION YEAR 2 DOCTOR

Presenting a piece of work in front of an audience can be a challenging and daunting experience for anybody. The most charismatic professors rehearse presentations for hours and sometimes days before giving them. A presentation is both artificial and show-like and, unless you are a rehearsed performer, one is not used to being in front of a group of people (albeit knowingly) who are scrutinising your every move. Therefore, it is normal to experience apprehension, anxiety or even fear. That being said, some experienced presenters seem at great ease every time and to the observer they do not show a flicker of anxiety. Although it may seem innate (and perhaps it is for some people), you can be assured that anyone can reach this stage with the right tips and hard work. Over time, a skilled practitioner learns various tricks and gains the experience needed to captivate any audience.

This chapter will take you through the various elements of what most people regard as the 'perfect' presentation, while expanding on the process that goes into presenting your work at a meeting or conference, including both poster and oral platform presentations.

THE PERFECT PRESENTATION

Everyone probably has a slightly different opinion of what the perfect presentation is and this is understandable. It is easy to find differences between two equally excellent speakers – one may be funny, ebullient and energetic while another may convey conviction, stability and wisdom. This is not to say that any of these adjectives are better than others; just that there is no 'perfect' presentation style, only *your* best presentation style. The audience usually dictates what qualities the presenter utilises, but the commonalities are also striking between different settings.

For excellent speakers, the most important aspects of presenting are to be articulate and clear. This may be obvious but it a very important part of presenting in front of a group of people: ensure each and every word is understood. You only have to think back to a university lecturer and how much strain it would have saved you if he or she would have only projected to the whole room rather than mumbling to him- or herself for an hour. Additionally, every sentence that a good presenter speaks builds on something he or she has said before to create a coherent story. Moreover, a good speaker is able to relate to his or her audience by either the things he or she says (i.e. language – by using colloquialisms or professional terminology) or the actions he or she performs, and so the speaker becomes engaging. Finally, it is the content that can separate the good speaker from the rest. Sometimes, at medical conferences, there are many speakers who are exceptional and the decision for a prizewinner may be the one who individual judges think had the most important content. Although this may be out of your hands with the research project you are given or the results that you may have from your project, you can always do things to make your presentation topical.

CHOOSING A PROJECT

It is not a joke that hard work will pay off. Although being in the right place at the right time can provide you with the connection that results in a publication for little work, you can shape your success at medical school with good preparation.

This begins by researching potential supervisors and projects that are suited to your interests. You will find that some researchers may hold prominent roles at your university but are relatively inactive academically, while others may publish every month yet fly under the radar. All is revealed on PubMed. Therefore, contact several people by email or directly and assess what is good for you and be prepared for meetings with them too. Be sure to look up information about what the researchers are doing with their work and what you find interesting. Remember, if at first you don't succeed, try again – you may spend several months and many emails and meetings before getting involved with a viable project.

Most people agree that getting something for your hard work is a must, and so you should aim for at least a poster abstract submission for every project that you undertake. It is also important to let your supervisors know if that is what you want. Some of them may even be keen to let you in on other projects if they see that you are enthusiastic.

CREATING A PRESENTATION

Before creating your poster or presentation it is important to have an idea of what you and your supervisor would like to showcase on it. Ask your supervisor to show you previous posters that he or she may have supervised in the past so that you can get an idea of the format that is expected. If not, you can still follow the usual section breakdown of a paper (introduction, methods, results, discussion, conclusion), putting the sections in separate boxes. Two or three illustrations will also be helpful for an observer. A sample poster is shown in Figure 18.1. A similar approach can be used for a presentation; you should remember to keep the text on each slide concise and to the point. Although it is tempting to go up in front of a crowd and read from a slide, doing this may not give you the best of scores for a prize later on if this is what you want.

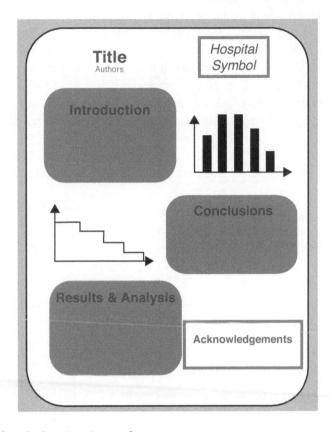

FIGURE 18.1 A typical poster at a conference

FORMAT OF POSTERS AND PRESENTATIONS AT A CONFERENCE

Posters and oral platform presentations at a conference will run according to an itinerary that should be available to all speakers and delegates a few months before the event. This will tell you whether you are scheduled first thing in the morning or late in the afternoon and also if you are required to be at another venue to present your research. It is important to read this well in advance of the date you are required to make the necessary travel arrangements. It can be beneficial to ask your supervisor, medical school, deanery or hospital trust if they have allowances for students or trainees to present at conferences, as you may benefit from this financial assistance.

You will normally be required to present for around 10–15 minutes at a conference, with the last 2–5 minutes reserved for questions. Therefore, it is important to focus on filling the time when you are presenting precisely, so that everything runs flawlessly and you are able to focus on clarity and conveying the core messages of your presentation to the audience. Although there may be many stems to your project it will be necessary to simplify it for the sake of a presentation.

There are some tips that are specific to a poster or PowerPoint presentation that need to be mentioned, as these are very important for first impressions that the audience and the judges see. Make sure that you do the little things right, such as choosing a background that is not too garish and using a font that is legible from the back of the presentation room. Also, make sure that the slides are sized proportionally to one another so that the final product appears to be produced professionally rather than a last-minute job. Make sure every diagram and table is clearly and consistently labelled so that there is unity to your presentation. Some people also choose to script their entire presentation and memorise it before presenting. Although this may seem artificial, it is highly recommended for inexperienced presenters to use this method, as it reduces

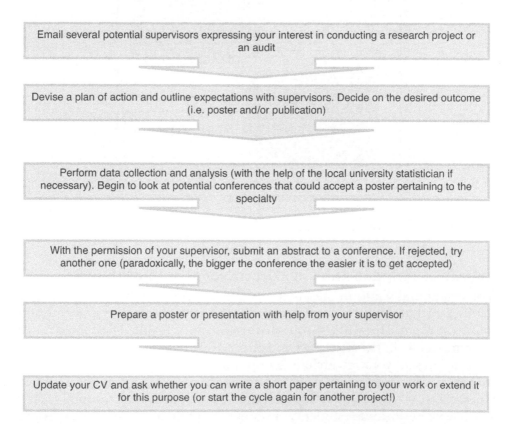

FIGURE 18.2 A flowchart of the expected sequence of events for presenting your work

or, for some people, eliminates superfluous words or pauses that a presenter would be prone to when in front of an audience.

Ideally, your presentation should be completed 2–4 weeks before the conference and you should be rehearsing it very frequently between then and presentation day. When you begin to get comfortable, start presenting to your colleagues, friends and the project supervisor. The less you to have to strain and think while you are presenting on the big day the better, and you will be less likely to make mistakes. If you do not want to memorise an entire monologue, then it is highly recommended that you memorise at least the beginning and the end, as it will make you feel at ease once you start and will also ensure that your presentation ends naturally.

You should anticipate any questions that an audience member may ask you. Depending on whether you are at a specialist conference or at a student's conference you will be asked at least one question. Your supervisor will be able to guide you and reveal any weaknesses in your study but it will be your friends who will tell you about anything that is unclear or that could be easily mistaken to the layperson. It is also worth knowing if any senior members who were involved in your project will be attending, as you can deflect any difficult questions to them.

Figure 18.2 shows the expected sequence of events while working towards a presentation and beyond.

ON THE DAY

The day before your presentation you should be very well rehearsed. Plan your journey to the area and make sure you have the necessary documents in order to register. Wake up early and have a good breakfast and dress smartly At this point it is advisable to go over your presentation one last time, just so that you are sure you know everything that is coming up – this is more to calm your nerves than to practise, as by this point your presentation should be well honed. Many conferences have equipment that is identical to that of the auditoriums, enabling you to check how things will look while you are presenting, ensuring you don't get any nasty surprises at the crucial moment.

While you are waiting for your presentation time to be announced, make sure to roam about and see what other presenters were able to accomplish, as this is a great time to know how far you can aim for any future endeavours you have planned (and also how much better your project may be!). When the time comes, go up and give it your best!

AFTERWARDS

After finishing your presentation, it always feels as if a huge weight has been lifted off your shoulders. Take a seat and enjoy the occasion. Even if you think it has gone badly, think about the positives that you can use from the experience. Add this experience to your CV; if you do not have a CV yet, create one, because this is a major accomplishment worth listing on it. It is also worth a point in your Foundation school or specialty training applications that can separate you from other candidates.

It is important to remember that the simple things often have the most impact and good preparation always goes a long way.

Section 5

The selection process and interviews

Gaining entry to medical school involves possibly the toughest competition ratio you will experience in the whole of your career – so if you are reading this after succeeding at getting into medical school, it is all downhill from here on in! However, while the competition ratios may be lower, there are still many positions that have ferocious competition, although do not be put off applying, for someone has to get accepted for the post – why not you?

Understanding the application process is vital to succeeding: 'forewarned is forearmed'.

This section will describe to you the different processes you may experience in your application. Not all selections will utilise all of these methods, with some favouring selection centres and others preferring a more traditional 'portfolio and interview' method. However, being au fait with the different techniques used for applications means that you are well prepared, whatever comes up. The main topics covered here are the 'selection centre', interviews and, most important, what to do if it all goes 'wrong'.

CHAPTER 19

Selection centres

Mr Mark Cookson and Mr Michael Ghosh-Dastidar

INTRODUCTION

As part of the evolution in medical training and application services, there has been a move towards national application systems and the use of selection centres. After shortlisting, candidates are invited to a selection centre where they compete for the positions offered.

The benefit is a standardisation of the process, aiming to produce a fair and transparent system. Current evidence supports the hypothesis that selection centres are a good method for accurately determining the best candidates for the careers applied. They not only provide an opportunity for traditional assessment via interview techniques and panels but also can often include OSCE, clinical, practical or situational judgement stations. Generally, candidates are marked by several assessors on a number of tasks or scenarios throughout the day.

The scope of this chapter is to familiarise one with:

- why they have come about
- what to expect
- how to prepare.

Additionally, this chapter provides some further sources of information.

It should be noted that selection centres vary according to region and specialty and one should check all documentation available from the specific centre once this is known.

HISTORY

Following the Tooke review in 2007, a move towards 'specialty tailored assessments at selection centres' was recommended.

Each specialty has gone on to develop their process to try to predict the best candidates for the post. Overall the crux of this change is aimed at trying to make things fairer – remove individual bias and select the best candidates for the jobs based on merit and ability to perform when required.

The aim is to try to select candidates who will have a long and fruitful career in their chosen specialty. It is now accepted that good grades at medical school do not determine whether one has the characteristics necessary for all career paths, as often other attributes are required. Each specialty has its own particular nuances and each person will need to try to glean what he or she enjoys and where he or she will excel.

WHY USE SELECTION CENTRES?

Previous application methods were considered:
- to be non-standardised
- to be region specific
- to be oversubscribed – affecting quality of assessment
- to have fewer assessors involved.

These were, therefore, subject to criticism on lack of transparency, shortlisting quality and unfair discrimination and were subject to subsequent legal challenge

Many non-medical fields, including the civil service, armed forces and police, have adopted the use of situational judgement tests and selection centres. This has been as a result of large-scale meta-analyses that demonstrate a strong predictive value for selecting good-quality candidates and the fact that selection centres show improved validity over previous methods.

Selection centres aim to use exercises that assess across a breadth of criteria defined in the person specification; they adopt a multi-trait, multi-method approach.

Nationally coordinated recruitment systems have helped to reduce the number of repeat applications to different deaneries and to standardise the process. This in turn has helped to improve efficiency and the quality of shortlisted candidates.

WHAT TO EXPECT

General practice has really led the way on this but most specialties now have either implemented, or are in the process of implementing, their national recruitment process. Each specialty is looking for certain characteristics in their candidates, but overall they are all looking for good people and diligent doctors who are expected to progress in their chosen field.

It is beyond the scope of this chapter to describe each specialty and the approach required, but speaking to colleagues and peers as well as reading the person specifications and further information available via the deanery and college websites will be useful for this.

The following information, however, should be useful in your preparation.

Interview panel

Interview panels usually consist of three or four members, each with allocated topics to cover. These usually involve two to three stations, each lasting 10–15 minutes (don't fret about this time – when you are there, it usually seems much quicker).

Most interview questions are designed around the person specification of the job, which in turn is linked to the GMC's *Good Medical Practice* guidelines. Therefore, it is important that trainees familiarise themselves with these guidelines before interview.

Potential assessment stations include:
- clinical judgement
- portfolio
- prioritisation
- presentation
- communication
- simulation
- practical skills
- ethical/professional – integrity
- written or data interpretation test
- management/leadership
- group interaction
- psychometric tests.

Please note this list outlines a selection of stations that may or may not be used and each specialty will have its preferred areas to cover.

Overall the selection centre is considered to be a broad-based assessment and assessors will be looking at the following attributes:
- commitment to specialty
- communication skills
- teamworking ability
- leadership
- time management skills
- situational judgement
- integrity
- initiative.

Presentation

You may be required to prepare and perform a presentation. This is usually allocated a limited time. The key is to remain calm and be strategic. Remember, everyone else has the same time – just be as effective as you can.

Key points are outlined as follows.
- Everything required will be provided.
- Read the brief very carefully and more than once.
- Look at the information and tools provided and make an initial plan:
  > allocate time and resources efficiently and appropriately.

- Try to use multiple methods of presenting your information (e.g. use diagrams if appropriate).
- Be concise and informative but stick to the time limits – they are strict limits.
- Speak clearly and deliver to the audience when presenting.

Simulation

Some assessment centres use simulated patients to judge a range of skills, but not just clinical abilities. Surgical application centres are likely to include practical or skill-based stations, but remember they are also assessing your ability to remain safe despite the pressured conditions.

Effective communication is essential. Make sure you verbalise clearly and politely while providing clear and specific instructions. Introduce yourself to everyone and use other personnel who may be 'hanging around' to help delegate tasks appropriately. In clinical judgement sessions, always have a plan, review your patient regularly and remember to ask for senior advice or support when appropriate.

There is a very useful DVD, *Selection Centres for Specialty Training*, produced by Health Education South West in conjunction with the Association of Graduate Careers Advisory Services. It is highly recommended that you watch this to get an idea of what goes on and how to deal with some scenarios effectively (www. agcas.org.uk/agcas_resources/37-Selection-Centres-for-Specialty-Training-second-edition-DVD-and-streaming-licence-).

PREPARATION

Preparing for the selection centre day can be the most important preparation of your entire career; do it well and you have given yourself a great chance of succeeding, do this poorly, and you will have to make up for being tired, hungry or ill-prepared for interview questions. The basics include finding out journey times, arranging accommodation, collating and printing out paperwork, organising your portfolio and making sure you are as prepared as possible.

Be nice, be yourself and always maintain a positive attitude and outlook. As well as preparing for what you may be asked in an interview, make sure you have a plan for food and that you are well rested for the day.

It is of the utmost importance to look clean and smart and to make sure your hands and fingernails are immaculate, your clothes are freshly washed and pressed, and your shoes are polished.

When answering questions, be sure of your answers or decisions, but do not appear aggressive or arrogant and try to be aware of your body language and maintain a natural level of eye contact. Overall, be polite, remain calm and be safe in your actions – nothing is better at getting a bad score than an unsafe answer to a clinical question!

Ensure you get plenty of interview practice. Discuss the common topics with colleagues, practise new questions and articulate your sentences in advance of the day. Have a message or structure to your answer and be succinct – don't just ramble on.

As well as interview practice, make sure you get lots of scenario practice. Research the common scenarios, understand what is expected in the different types of stations and plan how you will maximise your potential in each, even if this is just a basic structure which you can embellish on the day, depending on the specific question or scenario.

Figure out what skills they are assessing in the specialty by reading the person specification and make sure you can demonstrate evidence of these skills with support from your application and portfolio. Make sure you know your portfolio inside out, as this will show your career progression so far, as well as provide *evidence* of your competencies and your enthusiasm for the specialty. The importance of this cannot be understated, as without evidence it is assumed that the content is not reliable enough to be classed as suitable for inclusion in the assessment criteria.

Other things to research include answers to the core questions such as 'Why that specialty?' and 'What can you bring to this specialty?' Make sure your research involves speaking to current trainees in the specialty and ensure you are up to date by reading journals, especially the core journals for your specialty and at least one of the 'Big Four': the *Lancet,* the *BMJ,* the *New England Journal of Medicine* and the *Journal of the American Medical Association.*

Remember to start early; doing things at the last minute just makes you stressed, less able to focus on your goals and look a bit silly. As the old saying goes:

Fail to prepare, prepare to fail.

This is your chance to show your quality and commitment to what you intend to do for most of the rest of your life! Showing up unprepared says a lot and certainly will not benefit you.

It is crucial to be personable and not to alienate yourself. Ultimately, you want the assessor to think you are someone he or she could work and get along with but also that you would be reliable, get the job done and be trainable.

Do not be argumentative, and always discuss ideas or evidence in a way so as not to offend – that is, maintain humility even when you feel you may have further knowledge. Never forget to maintain respect for your assessors. Have a framework for your answers – sometimes it will be appropriate to use the STAR technique.

S = Situation: be concise and informative

T = Task: brief outline

A = Action: what exactly did or would *you* do?

R = Result: what was the outcome of *your* action?

You will be advised what documentation you will be required to bring to interview, but the list will most likely include at least the following:

- portfolio (including CV)
- original proof of identity (e.g. passport or photo ID)
- evidence of citizenship or eligible immigration status
- original and photocopy of your GMC certificate
- original and photocopies of your qualifications.

FURTHER READING

- www.mmc.nhs.uk
- www.medicalcareers.nhs.uk
- www.bmjcareers.com
- Royal college and deanery websites

CHAPTER 20

Best approach to interviews

*Dr Samantha Fossey and
Mr Charles Zammit*

Preparation is key to success at interviews and should start as you are preparing your written application.

An application timeline will be published for each specialty, normally by the coordinating deanery, which varies from year to year. The Modernising Medical Careers website provides information regarding which deanery is coordinating what specialty. Pencil in the dates for interviews so that you can swap on-call commitments and ensure you have adequate time to prepare. Most important, try to ensure you aren't on nights immediately prior to the interview!

Start by familiarising yourself with the interview process itself and what you are required to demonstrate. This can be achieved by ensuring you have a clear understanding of what is expected of you and how you are assessed.

WHAT IS EXPECTED OF YOU: PERSON SPECIFICATION

Always study the person specification for the specialty you're applying for in detail. The person specifications provide a clear and explicit list of qualities they wish a trainee to possess. It is important that you present not only evidence for the qualities you possess but also an insight into areas in which you are deficient. In areas where you are lacking evidence you should demonstrate that you not only appreciate your deficiencies but also are proactive and have a plan in place to develop in this area.

Person specifications can be found on the Modernising Medical Careers website (www.mmc.nhs.uk).

HOW YOU ARE ASSESSED: INTERVIEW STRUCTURE AND CONTENT

Invest your time in gaining a clear understanding of the stations that will be included within the interview. Interviews will normally be no less than 30 minutes and consist of a combination of three or more stations.

Types of interview station include:

- portfolio stations
- clinical scenarios
- professional dilemmas
- presentation stations (*see* Chapter 18 for advice on presentations).

Each station demands a slightly different approach and knowledge. By knowing what stations to expect you ensure that you will not be surprised on the day and that you can anticipate what questions may be asked. The following paragraphs outline an approach on how to prepare for each of the interview station types listed.

Portfolio stations

Most interviews will contain a portfolio station. Essentially, you must prepare to be an interactive tour guide of your portfolio. If you fail to signpost your most significant achievements the interview panel may fail to recognise them. Subsequently, a significant proportion of your time should be spent in studying your portfolio so that you can quickly and succinctly guide the panel through your key achievements. If you structure your portfolio logically according to the person specification, it will facilitate quick and easy navigation of your portfolio and subsequently make it easy to demonstrate why you possess the required attributes.

Clinical scenarios

In most interviews, clinical scenario stations will be structured much like a case-based discussion. Consequently, you will be provided with a summary of a clinical scenario and then asked how you would approach the scenario. In some interviews (e.g. general practice) clinical scenario stations can be conducted as an OSCE, where you actively demonstrate how you would approach the clinical scenario by interacting with patients/actors.

In order to prepare for the clinical scenarios it is advisable that you refresh your memory of the recommended investigations and management of common emergencies within the specialty you are applying. This station aims to ensure that you not only have knowledge of common emergencies but also have a logical and safe clinical approach to acute scenarios. You can rehearse for these stations easily during your clinical practice by routinely justifying the reasoning behind your clinical decisions.

In order to demonstrate a safe and logical approach to acute clinical scenarios it is important you develop a generic structure to use when answering these questions. For instance, for most clinical-based scenarios it is appropriate for you to start with '*I would utilise an ABCDE* approach to assessment of the patient*', and then move through each stage in detail, expanding as requested by the interviewer. In these stations keep things simple. The aim is to demonstrate not only your knowledge base but also that you have a clear and structured approach so that when under pressure you will remain a safe clinician.

Professional dilemmas

Do not underestimate the value of drawing from experience. Basing your answers, both in the clinical and the professional dilemma stations, on how you have dealt with scenarios in the past ensures you are presenting examiners with an accurate portrayal of how you deal with these situations. It also makes your answer more dynamic and genuine. Take some time to reflect on clinical experiences that have affected you either positively or negatively – each has a lesson to be learnt. The focus of professional dilemma stations can be broadly categorised into two areas: difficult communication or difficult decision.

Examples of interview questions asked within each station category are discussed in the next chapter.

THE TRIMMINGS

Invest in a smart, professional and neutral outfit that you feel confident and comfortable in. Ensure the outfit is ready to wear 24 hours prior to the interview. Last-minute ironing and sewing adjustments are not conducive to minimising stress on the day of an interview.

Most deaneries will send clear pre-interview instructions; read these carefully! They will often request you to provide multiple copies of certificates. As a minimum, expect to be asked to provide copies of:

- original proof of identity (e.g. passport or other photo ID)
- original and photocopy of your GMC certificate
- original and photocopies of all qualifications listed on your application form (translated if necessary)
- evidence of citizenship or elibible immigration status
- evidence of skills in written and spoken English.

Failure to provide copies not only implies that you cannot follow basic instructions but also will result in you having to find a photocopier minutes before the interview! Know where the interview is to be held, at what time you are expected to be there and ensure you leave enough time to reach your destination in a timely manner. Aim to arrive at your interview 30 minutes prior to registration.

---

*A = Airway, B = Breathing, C = Circulation, D = Disability, E = Everything else (i.e. examination of other systems, such as abdomen or limbs, and review of bloods, imaging, and so forth).

CHAPTER 21

Example interview questions

Dr Samantha Fossey and
Mr Charles Zammit

PORTFOLIO

'Please tell us about your research experience.'
Depending on how much experience you have will determine how uncomfortable this question will make you. If you have research experience it is important to quickly and succinctly present your experience and how you have developed. If you have little research experience, recognise this fact but do not dwell on it. Smoothly and quickly move on to demonstrate knowledge of the research process and a commitment to gaining this experience.

Good answers will be balanced, highlighting your achievements while recognising an area for development. Always include a plan for how to further develop.

'Please talk about an audit or piece of research you are particularly proud of and why.'
Before going to interview it is important to highlight any audit or research on which you particularly worked hard and enjoyed. Selecting a piece that you worked on extensively and were passionate about makes it easier to talk candidly and passionately about a project while demonstrating an understanding of research process.

For each audit and research project within your portfolio you should be able to discuss what went well, what was difficult and how this was overcome, and what you have learnt in order to develop your research ability.

Within this question, if you select an audit it is a good idea to structure your description of the audit in the stages of the audit process in order to demonstrate understanding of the process.

'Please highlight a work-based assessment you found particularly useful.'
For every work-based assessment form that you include in your portfolio you should know how it demonstrates that you fulfil the person specification. Work-based assessments are not only a quantitative but also a qualitative way

of receiving feedback for your work. Subsequently, choose a work-based assessment that demonstrates development and final achievement of a high standard. Alternatively, select a work-based assessment with qualitative feedback that has influenced your professional development.

CLINICAL SCENARIOS

'You are an on-call core surgical trainee who has been called by nursing staff on a general surgical ward. The nursing staff are concerned about a patient who has undergone a Hartmann's procedure and has no urine output. Please talk us through how you would approach this situation.'

'On-call' clinical scenarios demand that you demonstrate an ability to prioritise tasks according to clinical need. In order to prioritise, you need further clinical information. It is also important to demonstrate your ability to delegate tasks appropriately, to ensure timely investigation and management of patients. For example, can the nursing staff cannulate/bleed while you are making your way up to the ward?

After demonstrating the aforementioned, you can move on to demonstrate your clinical knowledge. In answering any clinical scenario station, structure your answer by utilising an ABCDE* approach, in addition to taking a history and examining a patient. This demonstrates you are logical and safe in managing acutely unwell patients. As you move through assessment you should highlight immediate management interventions that you would implement as you go along; for example, (a) airway adjunct if the airway is compromised, (b) supplementary oxygen if low saturations or respiratory distress, (c) insert a cannula if inadequate venous access. Remember that you should not move onto the next stage if you have not successfully remedied an issue at the preceding stage.

After your clinical assessment it is common practice to list differentials. This also aids in justifying the investigations you are going to request.

In a post-operative patient it is imperative that you have a good handling of what operation they have had and when. Reading through an operation note provides you with a clear understanding of what has been done and highlights any intra-operative complications that influence post-operative course.

In this scenario you are being asked to assess an anuric post-operative patient. To ascertain the cause of this, you need to have a clear understanding of the patient's fluid balance state. Categorise causes of anuria into pre-renal, renal and post-renal. In simple terms, the vast majority of surgical patients will either have pre-renal (i.e. shock, dehydration) or post-renal (i.e. obstructive) causes of oliguria. Your clinical assessment of a patient should clearly reveal which category is the cause of the patient's anuria. Don't forget it is important to note the urine output trend; that is, has the urine output gradually tapered

---

* A = Airway, B = Breathing, C = Circulation, D = Disability, E = Everything else (i.e. examination of other systems, such as abdomen or limbs, and review of bloods, imaging, and so forth).

off or has it stopped abruptly? The latter would suggest a possible obstructive cause; is the catheter kinked? If the urine output has gradually tapered off it suggests a pre-renal or renal cause. In this scenario, if you are told the patient is hypotensive, tachycardic and spiking temperatures and day 10 post Hartmann's procedure then you would be highly suspicious of an abdominal collection causing septic shock resulting in anuria or oliguria. Low urine output management is determined by cause. For example, post-renal causes require intervention to relieve obstruction (e.g. catheter, ureteric stent or nephrostomy), while pre-renal causes require adequate fluid resuscitation.

Remember, being systematic and methodical in your response means that you appear to be a calm and professional person at times of stress and, most important, someone that the interviewer will be happy to leave alone at night looking after his or her patients – an excellent thing for the interviewer to be thinking.

'You are a core surgical trainee who has been called by ward staff regarding concerns about a gentleman who is continuing to bleed per rectum. Please talk us through how you would approach this situation.'
As mentioned earlier, 'On-call' clinical scenarios demand you to demonstrate an ability to prioritise tasks. The most important fact to ascertain in this scenario is the haemodynamic status of the patient. Additionally, if a nursing colleague is able to cannulate, it is important to establish large-bore access as soon as possible; alongside this, repeat bloods (including haemoglobin, clotting, group and save) should be sent.

You then proceed, as in the previous example, with an ABCDE approach. It is important to accurately assess a patient's haemodynamic status and to implement appropriate resuscitative measures in order to stabilise him or her. Don't forget catheterisation in order to optimise your ability to assess response to resuscitation.

After your clinical assessment it is common practice to list differentials. This also aids in justifying the investigations you are going to request. As mentioned in the previous chapter, it is important to revise the initial investigation and management of common surgical emergencies so that you can confidently discuss such scenarios. However, it is important to remember that the majority of marks gained in these scenarios are for the use of a safe and logical, ABCDE approach rather than your knowledge base in itself.

'You are a ST1 paediatric trainee who is clerking a 9-year-old boy who has fallen off his bike and is complaining of left upper quadrant pain. Please talk us through how you would approach this situation.'
Much like the previous scenarios, you need to utilise a logical approach – that is, history taking, examination (including ABCDE assessment) and initial management. This scenario tests your ability to assess a trauma patient as well as deal with issues specific to paediatric patients – for example, non-accidental injury. In this situation it is important you ascertain mechanism of injury; it is

likely then that you will discover he has fallen onto a handlebar in the area of his left upper quadrant. You are interested in mechanism of injury, not only in order to determine differentials but also as part of your assessment to exclude non-accidental injury.

The GMC provides core guidance regarding the protection of children and consent for both children and adults. Familiarisation with this guidance proves useful in discussions regarding these topics that may come up in the interview process. Guidance can be found online.[1]

PROFESSIONAL DILEMMAS

'A 15-year-old female patient who presented with right iliac fossa pain underwent a diagnostic laparoscopy, which demonstrated a right-sided ectopic pregnancy. While walking through recovery, her mother stops you to enquire as to what was found intra-operatively. The patient is still recovering from her anaesthetic and consequently has not yet been updated on how the operation went. How would you proceed?'

The GMC guidance referenced in the previous example provides adequate preparation for dealing with such a scenario. It is important to remember that the priority in this scenario is to maintain patient confidentiality. It is also vital that you recognise this would be a difficult scenario, and one that would require good use of clear communication. You have to balance assertiveness with empathy for a concerned mother. In such scenarios interviewers may push you to change your stance on the situation, making you feel cornered. If you have familiarised yourself with GMC guidance and stick to the advice therein, then you can be confident in your approach.

'You are a core medical trainee on the respiratory medicine ward out of hours tying up end-of-day jobs with your FY1 colleague. Your specialist registrar and consultant are not available. While on the ward you are approached by the matron and asked to talk to a relative of a patient who has been investigated for suspected lung cancer. The relative is frustrated and demands to talk to a doctor. How would you deal with this situation?'

It is likely that during your clinical experience you will have encountered similar scenarios. Prior to going to speak to a relative or patient you should always familiarise yourself with the clinical case so that you can answer questions honestly and also recognise the limitation of the existing clinical knowledge. Explain to the matron that you are happy to talk to the relatives but you will need to familiarise yourself with the case first. You can then either explain this to the relative yourself or ask the matron to explain that you will be coming to talk to the family after updating yourself with the case. Once you have familiarised yourself with such a case it is appropriate to find a colleague from the multidisciplinary team to accompany you (e.g. the matron). If the relative is being aggressive or abusive it is important to clearly and tactfully state to them that such behaviour is not tolerated within the NHS. If you feel that staff or patient safety is compromised then it would be appropriate to mention that you may call on security colleagues to assist in dissolution of the situation. The conversation should be held in an appropriate area (e.g. a quiet room) while maintaining safety – that is, you are accompanied by another staff member and have easy access to exits.

Prior to starting any information giving, it is important to ascertain the understanding of the individual with whom you are talking to ensure you provide information at an appropriate pace and level. If you are talking to a relative it is important to remember you need to gain the consent of the patient prior to any disclosure of information.

'In light of a change in training combined with the European Working Time Directive (EWTD) it is increasingly difficult to gain sufficient theatre time. Can you discuss how you will deal with competition for theatre time in order to ensure you receive adequate surgical experience?'
In order to prepare for such a question you should have a sound understanding of what is required from a surgical trainee. Collate information from existing trainees, clinical experience and taster weeks to inform you regarding what will be required of you. This demonstrates you have a sound understanding of what you will be required to achieve and that you have considered how to achieve it. To apply for surgical training you are required to collate a logbook of surgical experience. You can use this as direct evidence that you have an ability to maximise training and negotiate an appropriate level of surgical exposure and training according to your stage. It is important to recognise that clear communication and assertiveness with colleagues will assist in your ability to maximise your theatre time. It is important to appreciate that surgical procedures can be divided into a variety of stages; you may not be able to scrub and actively assist throughout a complex procedure but you could scrub, observe and therefore place yourself in prime position to volunteer yourself for closing skin, for instance. This conveys that you appreciate the training needs of others but are motivated to balance this with your training needs to achieve balanced training outcomes for the team.

'How do you think the EWTD has and will affect training within this specialty?'
This topic has been popular within interviews in various specialties. Subsequently, background reading on this topic is important for interview preparation. It will also reassure interviewers that you are aware of the wider environment in which you train. The website of the Royal College of Surgeons provides a comprehensive summary of the EWTD development and their response to its development.[2,3] The Royal College of Surgeons and the Royal College of Anaesthetists published a core report outlining solutions for maximising training in the context of the EWTD.[4]

'You are a core surgical trainee. The theatre sister approaches you and explains that, because of lack of bed availability, cases on your consultant's list need to be cancelled and the list re-prioritised. Your consultant and registrar are in theatre with a difficult

case and subsequently have not been made aware of this situation. How would you proceed?'

As a junior surgical trainee it is unlikely that your consultant would be happy for you to cancel lists without prior discussion with your senior team. Characteristics they are likely to value in a junior trainee are outlined as follows.

- *Recognition of their limitations*: it is possibly the most important trait in a junior doctor to understand when they require senior help. Getting this early can save lives. Demonstrating how important you deem patient safety as well as showing the humility of accepting your limitations, shows maturity and will ensure that you do not make mistakes by trying to act alone beyond your clinical competencies.
- *Initiative and insight*: it is important to appreciate that there are procedures or stages within a procedure where interruption would not be appropriate. Subsequently, attempt to prioritise the list while your registrar and consultant are overcoming the difficulty in theatre. It may be that by that time they will then be available to discuss the scenario.
- *Communication*: it is crucial to communicate with the multidisciplinary team in this situation. Clearly communicate to the theatre matron how you plan to proceed. She then has an understanding of how you plan to proceed and may be able to find an alternative solution (e.g. another consultant who can authorise cancellation).

REFERENCES

1. General Medical Council. *Good Medical Practice: explanatory guidance*. Available at: www.gmc-uk.org/guidance/ethical_guidance.asp
2. The Royal College of Surgeons of England *EWTD Timeline*, Available at: www.rcseng.ac.uk/policy/ewtd-timeline/
3. The Royal College of Surgeons of England. *European Working Time Directive (EWTD)*. Available at: www.rcseng.ac.uk/fds/nacpde/eea-qualified/ewtd (accessed 10 May 2014).
4. The Royal College of Surgeons of England. *Surgery and the European Working Time Directive*. Available at: www.rcseng.ac.uk/policy/documents/Surgery%20and%20 the%20European%20Working%20Time%20Directive.pdf/view (accessed 10 May 2014).

CHAPTER 22

When things don't go to plan

Dr Joseph M Norris

ACADEMIC FOUNDATION YEAR 1 TRAINEE

What do you do when life deals you awful cards? Do you give up? You could do, but this game is tough and if you want to make the most of your medical career, you're going to have to move on. This book is packed with impeccable advice from a host of well-informed individuals; embracing their suggestions will surely help you maximise your success. Unfortunately though, no matter how many tips and tricks you utilise, something, at some point, will go wrong. This is part and parcel of life as a human being. The fact that you are ambitiously pursuing an intense and tumultuous occupation will only make the likelihood of failure greater. Positions in the medical profession are undoubtedly still difficult to secure, despite recent plateauing of post-Foundation training competition ratios. That being said, setbacks along the way do not necessarily mean that you are a bad student or a bad doctor – not at all. Things go awry even for the very, very best. What truly matters is how you deal with these (perceived) catastrophes.

It is not the aim of this chapter to make a medical career seem so tough that failure and depression are inevitable and that hard work is futile. Nor should this chapter come across as some incarnation of a queasy, patronising self-help paperback! With any luck, you'll take something practical away.

An example of a horrendous situation that medical students occasionally face is given in this chapter as a case study. The resolution has been divided into five logical steps. Each step represents a set of emotions, thought processes and, most important, actions that must occur to overcome the given calamity. All being well, you will be able to adapt this approach to your own troubles, to help you make the best of the worst. While this example is focused on examination failure, there are myriad additional 'worst-case scenarios' that medical students and junior doctors face on a daily basis, including:

- scoring lower than predicted or expected on pieces of coursework, essays and exams in medical school

- failing pieces of coursework, essays and exams in medical school
- not meeting the innumerable deadlines expected during medical school
- being ranked lowly in your interquartile or interdecile ranking at medical school
- not being offered the first choice of deanery, hospital or specific job for the first job as a junior doctor
- rejection from the chosen core training programme
- not obtaining the specific desired core training job
- failing different sections of membership exams
- not securing any position on the chosen specialty training programme
- inability to get the specific desired specialty training job
- failing fellowship exams
- not attaining relevant fellowship placements.

CASE STUDY

This case study is designed to outline a nightmare faced by medical students each year. The steps provided are readily applicable to any unexpected negative situation that you might encounter in the future.

That's it! You've finished your finals. Probably the most stressful exams you will ever have to sit in your life. Five years of blood, sweat and tears have gone into them and they are finally over. Having just emerged from the final medical OSCE, pale-faced and dark-eyed, with more grey hair than you remember, you naturally ask yourself, 'How did that go?'

Oh dear! You forgot to suggest an intensive therapy unit (ITU) referral for that lady with neutropenic sepsis and you totally forgot to take an alcohol history from that depressed man. How did you manage that? It is totally natural for students to think about where they went wrong in the post-examination anti-climax period – and medics seem to enjoy ruminating over this more than any other students. Most of the time this is misplaced and students sail through with flying colours, despite those odd lingering doubts. But is this time different?

After a week spent testing your liver function and bronzing in the Grecian sun, you return to home to collect your results. Your friends manage to check their emails on the smartphones before yours comes to life. They squeal with delight – they made it through – they're doctors! Your phone buzzes and you open up your email:

Dear student, we regret to inform you that the examination board has concluded that you have not passed this component of the curriculum. The school office will contact you in due course.

Your stomach turns, intense nausea, sympathetic overdrive. How has this happened? You read the email more closely and it makes you feel worse. The inevitable thoughts and doubts that flooded your mind post-medical OSCE are for once founded in truth. You did fail the oncology station and you did fail the psychiatric station. Other sporadic errors throughout the examination collected and have resulted in an overall failure of the medical OSCE. And thus your finals. And medical school.

Step 0: Has it actually gone wrong?

One possibility is to make a quick and rough assessment. Very occasionally, the purported disaster is false, or in the very least, amenable to a quick fix. For example, sometimes a prompt phone call to a senior colleague may stop a crisis dead, before it becomes a reality. These situations are not really the focus of this chapter, hence this is 'step 0'. More often than not, you will have to genuinely deal with the circumstances and consequences, whatever they may be.

IN THE CASE STUDY

- Has the email been sent to the correct person?
- Can the exam be remarked?

Unfortunately, nothing can be done in our example. The final medical OSCE was failed, fair and square.

Step 1: Acknowledgement – acknowledging the event

The first real step in dealing with a bad situation is to acknowledge that it has happened. You have to realise that there are no time machines – you may want to be a doctor, but you will never be the Doctor from *Doctor Who*. There is no way of going back in time and fixing the books; what has happened, has happened. It is not helpful to deny it to others or to yourself. It can be difficult, embarrassing, upsetting and demoralising. No matter what the circumstances are, the sooner you can recognise that it has gone wrong, the better. Acknowledgement is pleiotropic in its effects. First, it can be cathartic, facilitating outpouring of emotion. Second, it promotes reflection and introspection. Third, and on a practical level, it enables necessary acts to occur, such as informing loved ones (to support you) and tutors (to guide you). Fourth, and finally, it allows for careful strategic planning to occur, regarding how the new future will be tackled.

IN THE CASE STUDY

Acknowledgement following failed finals must be one of the most painful things possible for a medical student. To see all of your colleagues relishing their success only makes the whole deal seem worse. The build-up, the work, the money, the time and the expectations culminate to make failure at the end of medical school a sickening blow, but true and honest acknowledgement is mandatory to move forward.

Acknowledging failure here is incredibly useful. It allows friends and family to provide support during the aftermath and it permits them to react appropriately. There is nothing worse than having an 'elephant in the room' – you can bet that everyone already knows, so it is sensible to acknowledge and admit it yourself. Acknowledgement would facilitate involvement from the medical school, for recap revision sessions and a resit OSCE.

Step 2: Reflection – identifying where things went wrong

Once you've had enough time to wallow, it is pertinent to move on to the next stage. While the 'catastrophe' is still relatively fresh within your mind, you need to identify exactly which areas went wrong. Take a piece of paper and a pen and gather the appropriate materials. These might be exam scripts, interview score sheets or marked portfolios. Then, either alone or preferably with a senior colleague, tutor or trusted peer, meticulously scrutinise the material, making a note for every occasion when something could have been done better. Again, this is a painful process, both emotionally and intellectually. It can be extremely valuable though, as it gives a comprehensible list to focus on during the 'recovery period' when amending the apparent disaster.

Interestingly, this exact process – retrospectively pinpointing problem areas – is a real and important part of medical practice. It is often done professionally, in complex medico-legal cases (that most doctors are likely to experience at least once in their career) and it is also done in patient safety departments, when trying to unravel serious incidents, to ascertain causality and direct future preventive measures.

IN THE CASE STUDY

OSCE examiners take notes on pro forma mark sheets and these are often readily available from medical schools, particularly in such circumstances as these. Obtaining these would be the first port of call in this step. Going over these carefully with a clinical or academic tutor would be essential to identify areas for future work. In this example, it seems that oncology and psychiatry may be good places to start!

Step 3: Planning – decide how this event will change your future actions

Having acknowledged the event and made a list of the causes, it is time to pause and make a plan about exactly how you are going to rectify the situation. Each point noted in the previous step must now be given an 'action plan'. This might involve gaining more clinical experience, buffing up certain areas of your CV or revising particular parts of your curriculum. Make sure every point has a practical solution and that you have the time and resources to put each one into effect. It is worth considering this carefully. There is little point saying that you will publish 10 original articles before your next interview in a couple of months – it simply won't happen. Lastly, it is pertinent to not let your weaknesses at the last failed juncture become your sole priority; make sure the rest of your CV and knowledge remains strong. It would be disastrous to let those slip.

While it could be argued that there is overlap between this step and the previous one, in actual fact, planning is a tremendously important process that warrants due respect. As well as planning for the short term regarding the logistics of solving each problem, it is worth planning for the longer term. The shock to this system that a 'worst-case scenario' can bring presents an apt time to think long and hard about your future hopes and dreams. It may be at this point that you decide to change tack (on various levels). Perhaps if the list you formed in step 2 is too formidable, or if the respective solutions are too challenging, you may decide that perhaps you don't actually want to be a neurosurgeon, or you don't really want to work in the centre of London – or (wait for it) you might not want to be a doctor. Remember there is nothing wrong with any of these viewpoints! It may dawn on you at this point that although things seemed bleak, they have provided insight that you would have otherwise lacked.

IN THE CASE STUDY

An OSCE revision timetable should be drawn up. This should be detailed and realistic, with adequate input from medical school and willing peers (as volunteer patients). Also, plans should be made for the remaining year. Can you begin your job as a junior doctor normally? Can you locum? (Not as an FY1, but in other situations this may be pertinent.)

Step 4: Action – turn your unexpected situation around

Often when things haven't gone as we initially wanted them to, we perceive ourselves in a worse situation because of this. This is natural and follows unfulfilled expectations. Now is the time to fix this. Having diligently planned your attack, it is then time to execute it. Arrange your carefully planned action points in chronological order. It is worthwhile to keep checking your progress to see that you are on track to achieving your goal, and this can be done with a tutor. At this point, you are likely to still feel raw from the initial insult and so will pour your soul into whatever it takes to turn your bad scenario around. This is fine, as these types of 'pushes' are responsible for success. Keep healthy though – do not allow your determination to harm your well-being. Sleep well, eat well and exercise. If you are able to do all of these things, then you will pass that examination or be given the fellowship that you desired, all being well.

IN THE CASE STUDY

Do the scheduled revision. Do it again! Practise on friends and family. Recap all of the old material. Then it should be time to resit the medical OSCE – and pass it.

Following this, the plans for the remaining year should be carried out, whether it means becoming a locum doctor or using the time wisely to amass relevant clinical experience and bolstering the academic side of your CV, such as with publications and presentations.

Step 5: Persistence – keep going!

Now that whole ordeal is over and you have realised that the world is not going to end, it is time to move on. There is little use in feeling regrets about mistakes (or supposed mistakes) that have been made in the past – only the future can be changed. Likewise, the experiences associated with these nightmare situations should not written off and whitewashed from your memory. First, you can use them to spur you on to further success. Failure tastes bitter and once you have had it you will not be keen to go through it again; so in future challenges, you might face them with more preparedness than you otherwise would have done. Second, such 'failures' can teach you practical lessons by highlighting weaknesses. If you had gotten in a mess because of poor organisational skills (not uncommon), buy a wall planner, get a good diary, get friendly with Post-it notes and use all of the functionality of your smartphone. Don't get caught out again.

IN THE CASE STUDY

Passing the resit OSCE marks the resolution of this dire situation, although it was humiliating to see colleagues of 5 years continue without you. Use the rest of the year wisely. Use the feelings of the event to prevent similar things occurring. In future, learn from this failure so that upcoming assessments, such as the membership exams, go more smoothly.

DO AND DO NOT IN DISASTER

When it all seems to have gone wrong, remember that in actual fact it probably hasn't. As well as following the five steps already outlined, there are several things that you should do and several things you should not do, to make the best of a bad situation.

Do

- Allow time for feeling sorry for yourself but make it a predefined, finite period. Hibernate, order takeaway pizza and give yourself the opportunity to wallow, but set a time limit. Unexpected 'failures' hurt and allowing these feelings to flow is natural, but only for a while. Engage with Google Calendar and set it to give you reminders on your smartphone: on a specified date in the near future, you must snap out of wallowing. You can book an appointment with a tutor or supervisor and use this as a deadline for you to aim for. You can view this as the beginning of the 'turn around'.

- Analyse your aspirations. Use a bad situation as an opportunity to assess yourself and your future. Are you heading down the path that you really want to? Medical disciplines can vary hugely and the earlier you decide whether a specialty is for you or not, the better. If you've been rejected from a microbiology PhD programme, it would be wise to think carefully whether you were really heading in the right direction. Do you really enjoy infectious diseases? Or do you find that you work better with children?
- Have a 'plan B'. Medicine is ferociously competitive. It shows perspicacity to have two or three potential career pathways planned out in your mind. While you might not rank them all equally, you should aim to have another route that you would be happy to follow if, despite your intense efforts, plan A does not come to fruition. Also, be prepared to deviate somewhat from your desired pathway. If you fail your membership exams and do not get onto core surgical training first time around, then why not take a laparoscopic fellowship abroad for a year. You'd come back stronger, refreshed and with a new perspective.
- Utilise everything at your disposal to get back on track. Get hold of as much material as you can. Locate exam transcripts and interview mark sheets and use them to plan your next move. Borrow or buy (don't spend too much money though) on guides for the exams that stand in your way. Speak to as many people as you possibly can for advice. Take some with a pinch of salt and listen closely to those in the know, such as programme leaders. Private coaching for medical careers or examinations is available, although use these cautiously, and only following strong recommendation from a friend. Become familiar with the abundance of Internet resources, such as the NHS Careers website (www.nhscareers.nhs.uk) and others. Harness everything you can find to win, but be tactful.
- Relish and celebrate success that you have had in the past. Always remember that you have come so far – it takes a lot to even get into medical school in the first place. Write down three achievements that you are especially proud of, such as an article that you have published or an examination in which you scored highly. Focus on this list during hard times and remember how success made you feel. This will bolster your self-worth and serve as a reminder that your current 'crisis' is merely a blip on the road to your ultimate goal.
- Seek guidance from professionals. Senior mentors who have been through the same rigmarole and professional medical career guidance services are ideal places to start when things get tough. They will have seen it all before and will be able to think clearly on your behalf, when you cannot.

Do not

- Make all of your decisions based on what those close to you say. Friends and loved ones will support you during difficult times, but the trouble is they will only say comforting things. Intriguingly, parents may be the worst; they will be so filled with pride by your plethora of other achievements that they cannot view your current hurdle objectively. Poor career moves can stem from friends' comments; for example: 'You're really good at woodwork – you should definitely go into orthopaedic surgery!' While such advice is pleasant, it may not always be well informed.

- Perceive 'failures' as being your individual fault. The number of competing medics continues to increase each year. Whether you are applying for a fellowship or a training post, or any competitive placement, you can be dead sure that the institution has had a 'record number of applications'. Indeed, in 2011 there were so many applicants to the Foundation Programme (many of them from outside of the UK) that 180 medical students were not initially allocated a job as a junior doctor. With so many applicants, interview panels and selection teams can pick and choose who they think is the best – on that day. There is always then going to be massive fallout. Those that don't make it shouldn't be downhearted, as on a different day, or at a different trust, or with a different panel, their luck is very likely to be different.

- Don't be hasty with your next move. When you've been knocked down you will probably feel like getting back on your feet again as soon as you can! If you have failed your membership exams, it may seem like the right thing to do to resit at the very next possible opportunity. This should be done with caution though. It may in fact be worth taking a little time to talk through the examination with a colleague to see where you need to improve your skills. If significant work is required, it would be wiser to bring yourself up to speed before investing more money in another potential examination fail. Similarly, if you do not get your dream job first time around, don't immediately settle for an available job in a specialty that you really don't like, just because it is easy to get. Take the time to consider your options. Don't set yourself up for a 40-year career of misery!

- Totally erase the ordeal from your memory. It is natural to want to forget about your negative experiences and there is nothing wrong with that. While you mustn't ruminate on them, it is pertinent to think about what can be learnt from your mistakes. If you fail to get a particular training post that you are aiming for, it would be worthwhile seeking out your interview score sheet. If you were unfortunate enough not to get an interview, it would still be wise to enquire to see what the minimum score was for interview. Conducting these painful post-traumatic exercises will help sharpen your application in the future and will help you ascertain accurately where you went wrong, and thus where you should improve.

APPRAISALS AND ANNUAL REVIEW OF COMPETENCE PROGRESSION

At your appraisal or ARCP, you will be required to show both that you have met the standards required to progress to the next level of training and that no one who has supervised your performance has any major concerns.

If you have a problem with your appraisal or ARCP, you normally get very detailed feedback and, barring major concerns about multiple aspects of your performance, instructions on how to address these concerns to enable you to progress. There are five 'outcomes' possible at review processes.

- Outcome 1: Satisfactory completion of training period
- Outcome 2: Inadequate progress; additional training time required – 6 months added to the Certificate of Completion of Training date (the date on which the certificate is awarded)
- Outcome 3: Inadequate progress; additional training time required – repeat year
- Outcome 4: Released from training programme
- Outcome 5: Incomplete evidence presented – additional training time may be required

The result for the majority of appraisals is either outcome 1 or outcome 5. Here you progress or have explicit instructions on how to do so in the time remaining between the appraisal and the date of your supposed progression. In the event of outcome 5, you simply have to provide evidence that you have addressed all concerns and, as a result, are suitable for progression to the next stage of your career.

Outcome 2 is not great, as it moves your Certificate of Completion of Training date back 6 months, but it simply means that you will spend a little longer in training before being able to become a consultant, which may allow you more time to become comfortable in your role – remember, you spend a long time as a consultant.

Outcome 3 simply means that you have not met the required standards and, in the view of the assessors, you will not do so given an extra 6 months of training. Therefore, you are required to repeat the year of training you have just undertaken. This is disheartening, but it also means that you can work with your clinical supervisor to address the problems highlighted in the appraisal. Often, this outcome is a result of long-term sickness or personal problems, so many people accept it with the mitigating circumstances and start the next training year with renewed enthusiasm.

Outcome 4 is the worst of the possible outcomes, but again, it is not the end of the world; it simply means that you have been released from this training pathway. You are still a doctor, you just need to apply for a different career within medicine. Often these come about in individuals who have applied for what they thought was their preferred career but which ultimately was not suited to them.

Whatever the outcome of your appraisal, the reasons behind the final decision are always conveyed, and remedial work clearly and thoroughly explained. The deanery and your educational supervisor are all working together to get the best out of you, while at the same time ensuring optimal and safe patient care. Therefore, if further training is needed, then this is for a reason. If you get anything other than an outcome 1, take the comments of the assessors on board, create a plan of action and follow through with it – you should be progressing at your next assessment with an outcome 1!

SUMMARY

Problems arise for everyone and at times they can seem overwhelming. Medicine is a tough field and as such there is a high likelihood of things going awry. The most renowned professor of surgery in Britain, Prof. Harold Ellis, freely admits to having failed his fellowship exams, and things at that time seemed bleak for him, but he rose from the ashes and so can you. It is to be hoped that this chapter has given you some practical suggestions about how to get through tough times, and how that when things seem to have all gone wrong, in actual fact, they might not have. Whenever you need to put the pieces back together, remember these steps.

- Step 0: Has it actually gone wrong?
- Step 1: Acknowledgement
- Step 2: Reflection
- Step 3: Planning
- Step 4: Action
- Step 5: Persistence

As well as this sequence, there are broader things that you should try to do and not do in a crisis. Allow time for introspection, but pick yourself up in good time and hit it twice as hard as you did the previous time. You will succeed. Sometimes, when things go pear-shaped, you may end up being pushed down a better road than the original one you had set out on. Lastly, remember: you are not alone.

Index

CPD with Radcliffe

You can now use a selection of our books to achieve CPD (Continuing Professional Development) points through directed reading.

We provide a free online form and downloadable certificate for your appraisal portfolio. Look for the CPD logo and register with us at: www.radcliffehealth.com/cpd

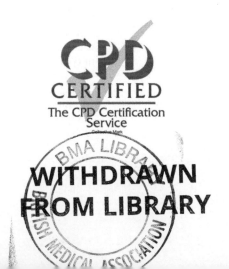